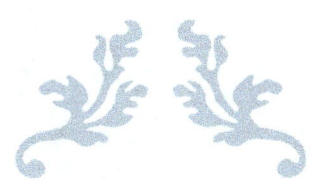

MEDITERRANEAN DIET SALAD RECIPES

DELICIOUS MEDITERRANEAN SALAD RECIPES FOR NATURAL WEIGHT LOSS, DETOX, AND HEALTHY LIFESTYLE

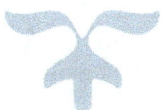

SANDRA RAMOS

Mediterranean Diet Salad Recipes

SANDRA RAMOS

Copyright - 2021 - All rights reserved.

The content contained within this book may not be reproduced, duplicated or transmitted without direct written permission from the author or the publisher.

Under no circumstances will any blame or legal responsibility be held against the publisher, or author, for any damages, reparation, or monetary loss due to the information contained within this book, either directly or indirectly.

Legal Notice:

This book is copyright protected. This book is only for personal use. You cannot amend, distribute, sell, use, quote or paraphrase any part, or the content within this book, without the consent of the author or publisher.

Disclaimer Notice:

Please note the information contained within this document is for educational and entertainment purposes only. All effort has been executed to present accurate, up to date, and reliable, complete information. No warranties of any kind are declared or implied.
Readers acknowledge that the author is not engaging in the rendering of legal, financial, medical or professional advice. The content within this book has been derived from various sources. Please consult a licensed professional before attempting any techniques outlined in this book.

By reading this document, the reader agrees that under no circumstances is the author responsible for any losses, direct or indirect, which are incurred as a result of the use of information contained within this document, including, but not limited to, - errors, omissions, or inaccuracies.

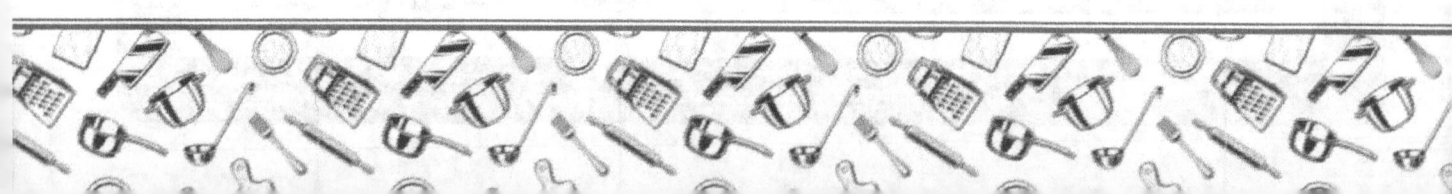

Table of Contents

INTRODUCTION 1

Chapter 1: Why this type of diet is the right for you? 5

Chapter 2: Your Mindset and this diet 9

Chapter 4: Exercise 15

Chapter 5: The recipes in this book 16

Salads 18

    Pesto Chicken Pasta Salad 18

    Asparagus and Artichoke Salad 19

    Chicken Spinach Salad 20

    Wild Rice Salad 21

    Tuna Salad 22

    Mediterranean Olive Salad 23

    Winter Vegetable Salad 24

    Tomato, Cucumber and Onion Salad with Mint 25

    Cabbage, Onion and Tomato Salad Greek Style 26

    Tuna Salad with Oranges and Pecans 27

    Asparagus Salad Italian Way 28

    Salad with Spinach and Cranberries 29

    Spinach, Peaches and Pecan Salad 30

    Cold Rice Salad 31

    Spinach Salad with Mustard 32

Spinach Salad with Pork Meat	33
Linguine and Shrimp Salad	34
Artichoke and White Bean Salad	35
Spinach Salad with Goat Cheese	36
Artichoke Salad vol.2	37
Seven Spinach Salad	38
Spinach, Berries and Curry Salad	39
Spinach Salad with Raspberries	40
Rice Salad with Artichokes	41
Ranch Salad	42
Strawberry Salad with Sunflowers	43
Anna's Salad	44
Tomato, Onion and Corn Salad	45
Pesto Chicken Pasta Salad	46
French Salad	47
Red Onion and Orange Salad	48
Watermelon and Avocado Salad	49
Asparagus and Strawberries Salad	50
Tomato and Basil Salad	51
Daiquiri Salad	52
Feta Artichoke Salad	53
Peanut Apple Salad	54
Onion and Strawberry Salad	55
Chicken Salad vol.2	56
Spinach and Pepper Jelly Dressing Salad	57

Feta, Couscous and Asparagus Salad	58
Pork and Walnuts Salad	59
Pomegranate Salad	60
Broccoli and Strawberry Salad	61
Blackberry Salad	62
Strawberry Ginger Salad	63
Chicken and Almond Salad	64
Asparagus Salad	65
Romaine Salad	66
Fruit Salad with Spinach	67
Cashew and Pecan Salad	68
Onion, Tomato and Cucumber Salad	69
Blue Cheese and Strawberry Salad	70
Mixed Greens and Gorgonzola Salad	71
Eggplant Salad	72
Mandarina, Orange and Gorgonzola Salad	73
SpringSalad	74
Orange, Asparagus and Endive Salad	75
Tossed Almond Salad	76
Cherry Vanilla Pear Salad	77
Lettuce Pear Salad	78
Arugula Salad	79
Creamy Orange Rice Salad	80
Beets in Orange Dressing	81
Bean Salad	82

Pepper Salad	83
Green Pea Salad	84
Krina's Tomato Salad	85
Tropical Tuna Salad	86
Greek Salad vol.1	87
Pesto Chicken Pasta Salad	88
Spinach Salad with Sesame and Ginger	89
Spicy Italian Salad	90
Steak and Spinach Salad	91
Palms Salad	92
Fresh Salad	93
Eggplant Yogurt Salad	94
Pear Salad	95
Chicken Salad with Pecans	96
Rice, Pecans and Chicken Salad	97
Honey Tenderloin Salad	98
Apple Salad	99
Pears and Ricotta Salad	100
Tarragon Salad	101
Blue Cheese and Pear Salad	102
Tossed Salad	103
Salad with Nuts	104
Feta Strawberry Salad	105
Red Potato Salad	106
Chicken Salad with Peaches	107

Orange and Mushroom Salad 108

Couscous Bacon Salad 109

Grape Salad 110

Chicken Salad with Lemons 111

Potato Salad 112

Quinoa and Lentil Salad 113

Summer Potato Salad 114

Seven Layer Salad 115

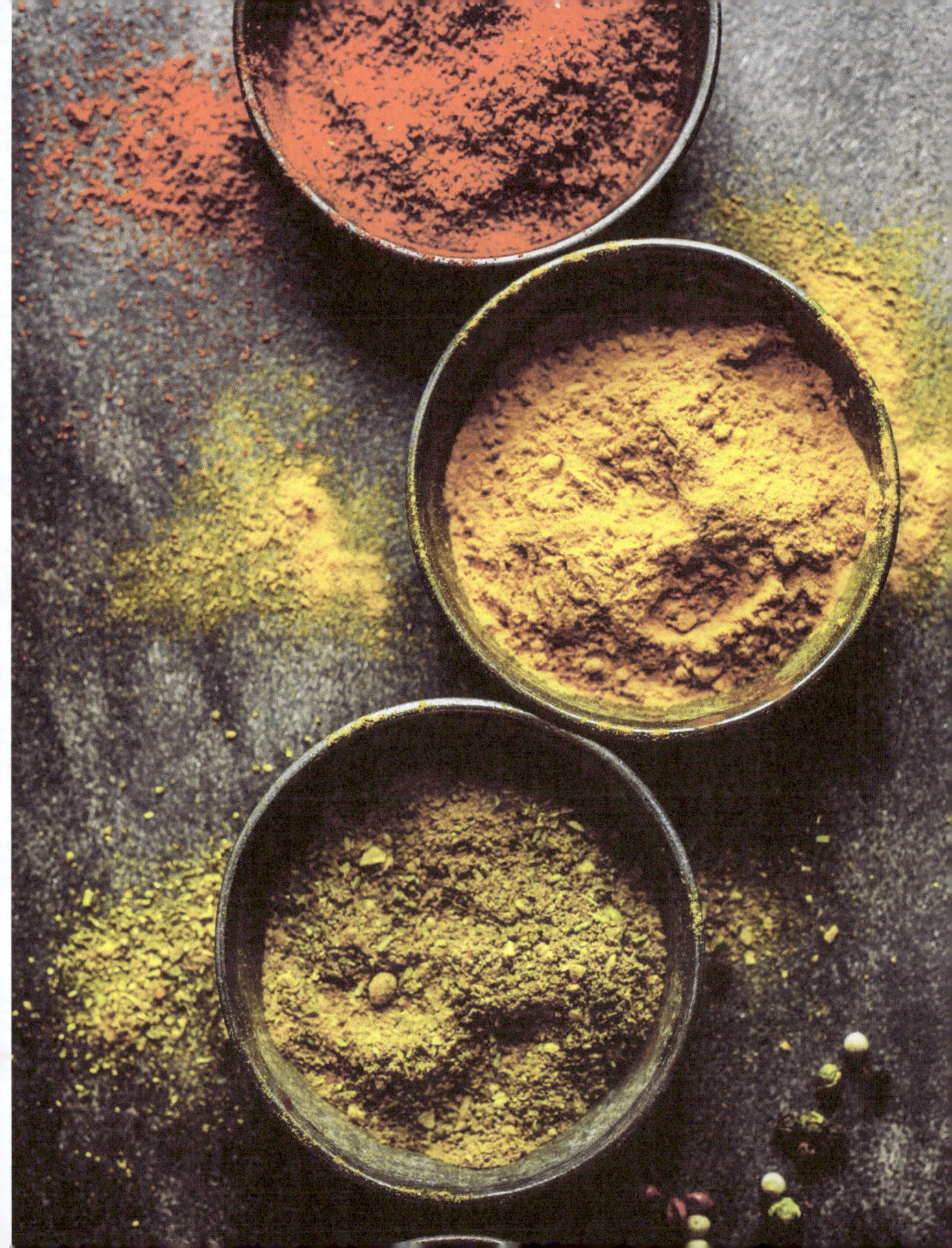

BOOK TITLE

INTRODUCTION

The joy that I am feeling right now cannot be explained. This is because you have chosen me and this book as a guide to a new path – the Mediterranean one. The Mediterranean diet is like no other diet in this world and this way of eating is offering many health and weight benefits.

Right after World War II, Ancel Keys, a scientist and his colleague Paul Dudley, later known as President Eisenhower's cardiac physician made a Seven Countries Study together with couple of their colleagues. They included people from United States and people from Crete – Mediterranean island. The study was testing these people of all ages and Keys implemented the Mediterranean diet in this study as well.

The 13,000 men came from Netherlands, United States, Greece, Italy, Yugoslavia and Japan and it was estimated that fruits, vegetables, grains, beans and fish are the healthiest ingredients ever. This applies even after considering the impoverishment of WWII. Interestingly this was also estimated at the start, imagine what else they discovered.

Among everything else it was discovered that Mediterranean way of food consumption can make one person lose and maintain healthy weight. Every chapter included in this book will reveal different story about this diet plan and how can you become able to change your eating patterns. Also, you will find out that Mediterranean diet plan gives extreme amount of energy and you will become motivated

Chapter 1: Why this type of diet is the right for you?

Simply because it contains healthy plant foods and it is low in animal foods. Unlike other diets, Mediterranean diet offers more seafood and fish. Seafood and fish are way better than any other meat and the benefits of them is visible after a week or two of constant consumption. Plus, Mediterranean recipes do not leave you hungry, you are full after eating for a longer period.

With constant exercise and fruits, vegetables, legumes, nuts and whole grains (everything that this diet is) you will become the best version of yourself without doubt. Also, you will learn how to perfectly switch bad ingredients with good ingredients. For example, instead of butter you will start using canola or olive oil. Instead of salt you will start using different herbs and spices. Print out the Mediterranean pyramid of foods and you won't regret it.

These recipes are family friendly and you'll be able to host and enjoy and host many gatherings with your friends as well because they are also friend friendly. Occasional glass of red wine is okay, so you are good to go.

HEALTH BENEFITS

Healthy fats are the key component when it comes to Mediterranean cuisine. Also, let's not forget about the most important thing this diet has – plant-based food. Yes, this diet does not remove many food groups, but the mixture of ingredients won't make you a single problem and you will learn what goes with what in time.

But let's elaborate on the health benefits a little bit more. It is scientifically proven that the Mediterranean diet is able to lower the risk of strokes and heart disease. Every patient that has used this diet style so far, has shown lowered levels of oxidized low-density lipoprotein or LDL cholesterol (the bad cholesterol which gets build up in your arteries and causes problems with your heart.

NO MORE HEART PROBLEMS AND STROKES

One of the main ingredients in the Mediterranean diet, extra virgin olive oil, contains alpha-linolenic acid and the Warwick Medical School delivered a study that indicated how olive oil is able to decrease blood pressure. Not only that but also the olive oil is able to lower hypertension because it keeps human arteries clearer and more dilated. Also, it makes the nitric oxide more bioavailable and you won't have problems with cholesterol levels anymore. Only if of course, you consume olive oil (extra virgin) on regular bases.

If you are feeling numbness, weakness, headaches, confusion, vision problems, dizziness or slurred speech do not worry no more. This diet helps and improves this condition together with the ultimate problem – strokes that are happening due to bleeding in the brain or blocked blood vessel.

IMPROVED VISION

Another thing that would improve after starting with this diet is your vision. This diet will help you prevent or stave off the risk of macular degeneration which happens to adults over 54. This disease brings blindness and occurs to over 10 million Americans. Imagine the benefit in here, imagine being victorious against something that is able to destroy your retina and remove the chance of clear vision. The vegetables this diet promotes, the green leafy ones have lutein and that lowers the chance of experiencing cataracts as well.

WEIGHT LOSS

You probably want to lose weight as well and the search for the perfect diet that will be able to provide you that is endless. Until now. This diet is also able to give you the chance to lose weight naturally and easily with nutrient rich foods. The focus in here is on healthy fats while carbohydrates are not that present. They are still here as pasta or bread of course, but their implementation is generally low. The healthy fats, protein and fiber will allow you to lose weight and at the same time will keep you satisfied. Thanks to these nutrients you won't have cravings for candy, chips or cookies no more. The vegetables that you'll consume will fill your stomach and you won't feel hunger for hours. You won't even experience spike in your blood sugar.

IMPROVED AGILITY

According to studies, 70 percent of the seniors who have risk of developing frailty or other muscle weakness lowered the factors of experiencing that by implementing this diet in their lives.

YOU'LL START ENJOYING NATURAL FOODS

This is probably the best thing that this diet brings because it is kind of a new characteristic that you'll develop. As previously noted, this diet is low in sugar and processed foods so its recipes will bring you closer to organic produced foods thus closer to nature. For example, this diet offers honey instead of sugar and this change is priceless.

IMPROVED ASTHMA SYMPTOMS

Another study which included children revealed that antioxidant diet is able to help them decrease their asthma symptoms and at the same time made them not like eating a food that is quite popular – red meat. Yes, this diet helps children to say no to red meat and yes to plant-based food.

NO MORE ALZHEIMER'S RISK

Those people that choose this diet plant without doubt lower their risk of getting Alzheimer's disease in the future. In fact, the latest study shows that getting Alzheimer's is reduced by 40 percent to those people that consume Mediterranean diet foods. Additional exercises are recommended in the process as well.

HELPS PEOPLE WITH DIABETES

Excessive insulin is controlled with Mediterranean diet. Not every diet is able to do this and not every diet can control blood sugar levels and control your weight at the same time. As I told before this diet is at the same time low in sugar and high in healthy acids. This makes a balance for your body and burns fat while gives you energy at the same time.

The American Heart Association reveals that this diet unlike other diets is low in saturated fat while high in fat. This keeps your hunger under control and delivers amazing weight loss results.

MEDITERRANEAN DIET HELPS YOUR BRAIN

Sugar is usually responsible for the highs and lows when it comes to your mood. This diet does not contain artificial sugar at all this your mood and overall brain health will improve as well.

THE WEIGHT LOSS JOURNEY

Planning breakfast, lunch or dinner is not hard, but the part gets tricky when it comes to snacking time. You should make something for yourself that contains from 150 to 200 calories. For example, you can choose apple, pear, grapefruit and a pinch of salt.

The path that this diet offers is the safest when it comes to losing weight. Everything is healthy here and there won't be bouncing.

But many people ask what happens when the time is stumbling on us and when we do not have time to cook the meals present in here. Well, I and this diet of course have a solution for you. Trust me you will like it.

- Fruit slices – pears and apples
- Nut butter – cashew butter, almond butter and more
- Dates and figs
- Tuna salad
- Crackers
- Greek Yogurt
- Olives
- Pitas
- Hummus

Chapter 2: Your Mindset and this diet

In order to remove the unwanted pounds, you have to set your mindset on it like never before. Do not think about that all the time, start thinking about something entirely else while you are focused on losing weight. Or in other words, keep yourself busy while you consume Mediterranean diet foods and you regularly exercise. Also do not expect quick fixes. Time is all you need and after successfully sticking to the plant you'll start to realize the change and how big it is.

To be sincere, the Mediterranean diet is the one thing that you have been missing for so long. You are already motivated I think so all you have to do is start. You already purchased this book, so you are on the right path.

Write down your reasons for starting this journey and every time you are feeling down, or you lack motivated read them out loud. Write down your goals as well. Start with something small and increase as time passes.

Another important thing that people usually forget are their surroundings. It is important for you to surround with people that are positive. Positive mindset regardless of what you do is important, especially when it comes to losing weight and changing something as diet pattern. This is how you'll become able to develop emotionally, healthy realistic goals (do not forget to set your goals first).

Focus on your sleep and develop a healthy sleeping pattern as well. Recharging and sleeping for more than 7 hours are essential when it comes to weight loss because you need extreme amount of energy and sharpness. Good energy and brain sharpness appear only when one is able to properly relax and recharge in the evening hours.

Chapter 3: Nutrition and Portions

Start being aware of the things you consume now. Develop your management skills and stick to the guidelines that this book gives. What to consume? Well start with:

- Vegetables – raw and leafy
- Fruit
- Legumes
- Grains (one slice of bread is allowed)
- Dairy
- Meat
- Potatoes
- Nuts

This is the food you must start combining and portions that include these ingredients will make you set and ready for reaching your goals.

This is a sustainable diet so you won't have serious problems, but I will be lying if I say that cravings won't appear. If you successfully understand your cravings, you'll remove them and soon be proud of your dietary success. Remember, cravings for certain foods indicate need of something entirely else, something that your body is need of.

So, the adjustments that you have to make regarding the cravings are:

- Remove salty cravings with couple of nuts or seeds because your body want silicon.

- Remove fatty and oily foods with spinach, broccoli, cheese and fish because your body wants calcium and chloride.

- Remove sugary foods with chicken, beef, lamb, liver, cheese, cauliflower and broccoli because your body wants phosphorous and tryptophan.

- Remove chocolate cravings (this is the hardest one) with spinach, nuts, seeds, broccoli and cheese because your body wants magnesium and chromium.

You also have to:

- Learn how to recognize every healthy ingredient on the labels. Take back everything that does not look good to your or that indicates that there are many artificial preservatives present.

- Check your serving size.

- Always calculate your calories intake

- Consume food rich in calcium, iron, fiber, vitamin A and vitamin C.

Do not consume:

- Added sugar or foods like candy, soda, ice cream and more.

- Refined oils – soybean oil, canola oil cottonseed oil and more.

- Trans fats – margarine, soda, processed meats, beverages, table sugar and more.

- Processed meat.

- Refined grains.

Foods that you should consume:

- Seafood and Fish: Mussels, clams, crab, prawns, oysters, shrimp, tuna, mackerel, salmon, trout, sardines, anchovies, and more

- Poultry: Turkey, duck, chicken, and more

- Eggs: Duck, quail, and chicken eggs

- Dairy Products: Contain calcium, B12, and Vitamin A: Greek yogurt, regular yogurt, cheese, plus others

- Tubers: Yams, turnips, potatoes, sweet potatoes, etc.

- Vegetables: Another excellent choice for fiber, and antioxidants: Cucumbers, carrots, Brussels sprouts, tomatoes, onions, broccoli, cauliflower, spinach, kale, eggplant, artichokes, fennel, etc.

- Seedsand Nuts: Provide minerals, vitamins, fiber, and protein: Macadamia nuts, cashews, pumpkin seeds, sunflower seeds, hazelnuts, chestnuts, Brazil nuts, walnuts, almonds, pumpkin seeds, sesame, poppy, and more

- Fruits: Excellent choices for vitamin C, antioxidants, and fiber: Peaches, bananas, apples, figs, dates, pears, oranges, strawberries, melons, grapes, etc.

- Spices and Herbs: Cinnamon, garlic, pepper, nutmeg, rosemary, sage, mint, basil, parsley, etc.

- Whole Grains: Whole grain bread and pasta, buckwheat, whole wheat, barley, corn, whole oats, rye, quinoa, bulgur, couscous 18

- Legumes: Provide vitamins, fiber, carbohydrates, and protein: Chickpeas, pulses, beans, lentils, peanuts, peas

- Healthy Fats: Avocado oil, avocados, olive oil, olive oil products and olives

- Beverages: Water and tea

- White meat: Consume them but remove the visible fat and skin

- Red meat: You can consume lamb, pork, and beef in small amounts

- Potatoes: Prepare them with caution but consume them because they are excellent source of potassium, vitamin b, vitamin c and fibers.

- Desserts and sweets: consume cakes, biscuits and sweets in extra small amounts.

There is one thing that you can implement that will make your journey even more beautiful – spices and herbs! Traditional Mediterranean diet is filled with different spices and herbs and each has a different health benefit! Believe it or not herbs and spices are able to do that and that is one of the main reasons why people implement them in their diet. Here are the spices you must include and the benefits they bring:

- Anise – improves digestion, reduces nausea and alleviates cramps.

- Bay leaf – treats migraines.

- Basil – aids digestion and reduces anxiety and stress.

- Black pepper – promotes nutrient absorption and speeds up your metabolism.

- Cayenne pepper – increases metabolism and controls your appetite.

- Sweet and spicy cloves – relive pain, gum and tooth pain. Also, kill bacteria, fungal infections and aid digestive problems.

- Fennel – improves bone health.

- Garlic – improves blood sugar levels and helps you lose weight.

- Ginger – serves as diuretic and increases urine elimination.

- Marjoram – promotes healthy digestion and fights type 2 diabetes.

- Mint – treats nasal congestion, nausea, dizziness and headaches.

- Oregano – treats common cold and reduces infections. It also relieves menstrual pain.

- Parsley – improves your skin, prostate, dental health and blood circulation.

- Rosemary – increases hair growth, reduces stress, inflammation and improves pain.

- Sage – improves your digestion problems.

- Thyme – has antibacterial properties.

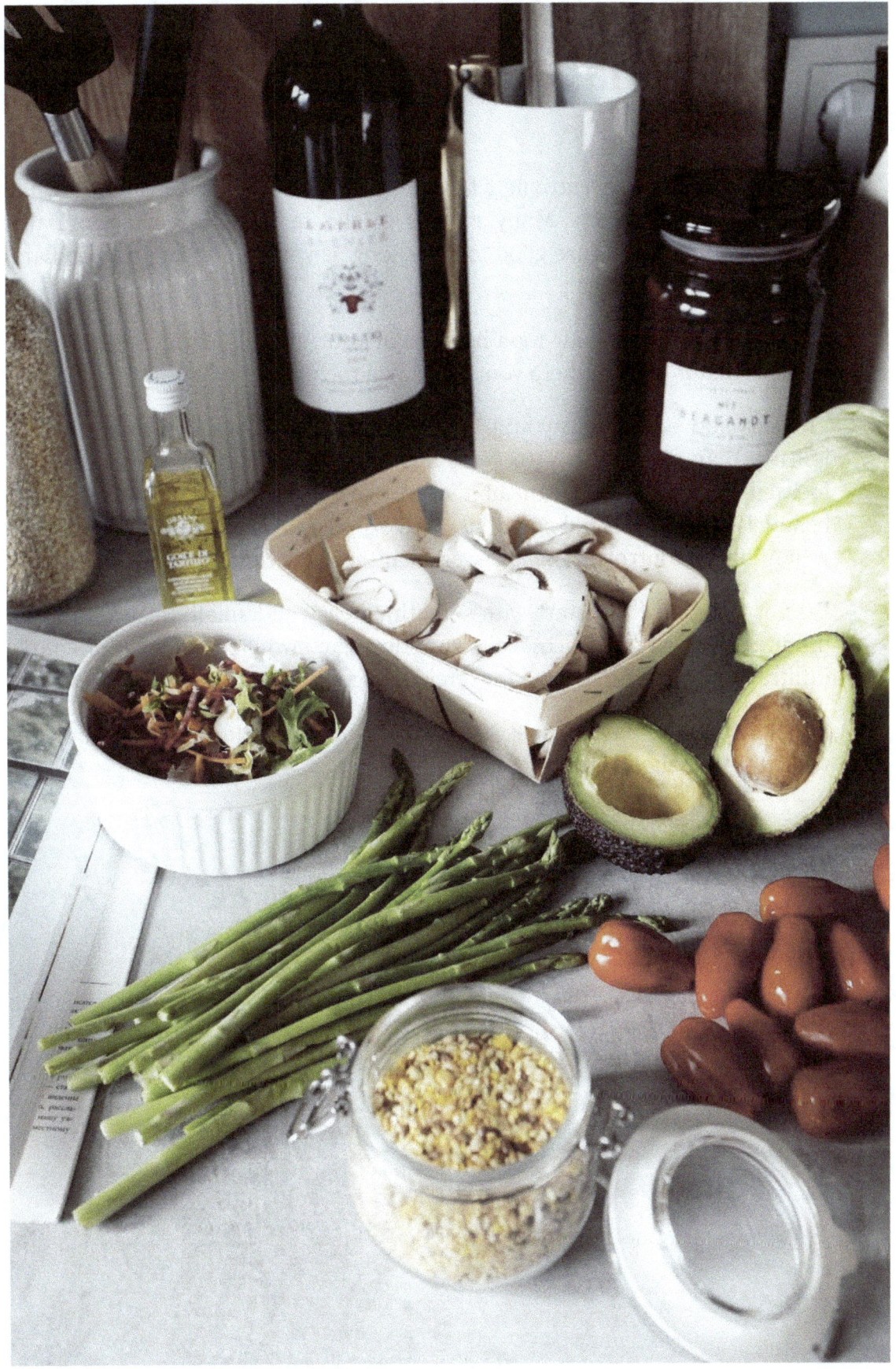

Chapter 4: Exercise

Mediterranean diet is extremely flexible, and you won't have problems while being out with friends. Many recipes in the restaurants come from this particular diet so, you are good to go as long as you do not eat junk food and food that is high in sugar.

Eat slowly and chew your food better. Put your utensils down between bites because that is going to help you slow down the process of eating.

The tips above will help you a lot, but nothing will help you more in this journey than exercising. Two years ago, one scientific research that mainly focused on the Mediterranean diet revealed that this diet is extremely beneficial and gets its full potential when exercise is included. So, to keep your weight under control and to lose weight at the same time you must exercise.

Do not force yourself, start with something easy and small. Spend 30 to 60 minutes daily on that part. Walk, run, do yoga, swim, ride a bike, or simply infiltrate yourself into a regular exercise program online or in a gym near you.

Regular physical activity does not improve only your look, it also improves your strength, mood and balance.

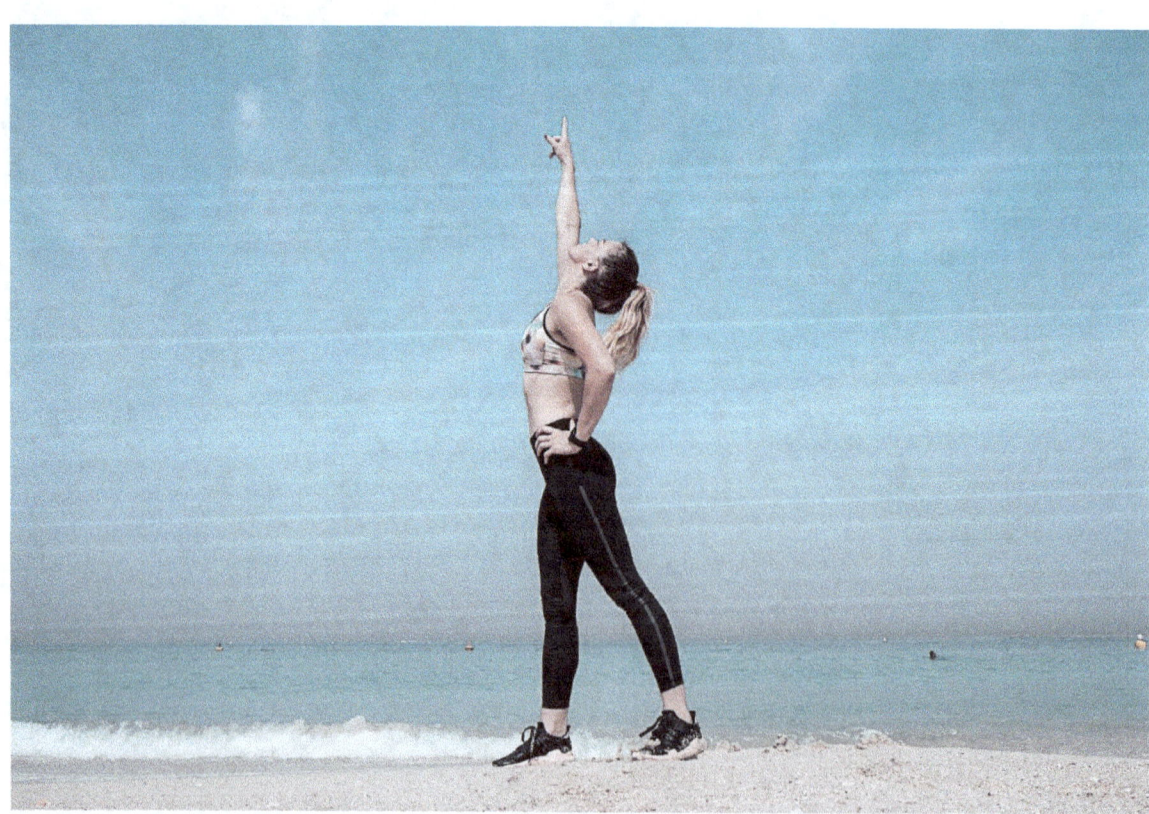

Chapter 5: The recipes in this book

This book contains 500 recipes in total. Each recipe is designed according to the rules Mediterranean diet has. Every recipe is healthy, and every recipe should be made with the best ingredients available – the organic ones. There is also a section for vegans and vegetarians. We wanted to include every person possible in this journey because this journey is all about health and improving yourself and the way you eat. At the bottom of this book you will find a meal plan that we think is going to help you a lot in the few first months. The start won't be that hard, but it is going to be challenging I must admit.

The cooking skills

It is important to know that the Mediterranean do not require hours and hours in the kitchen. The way these recipes are prepared is easy and convenient.

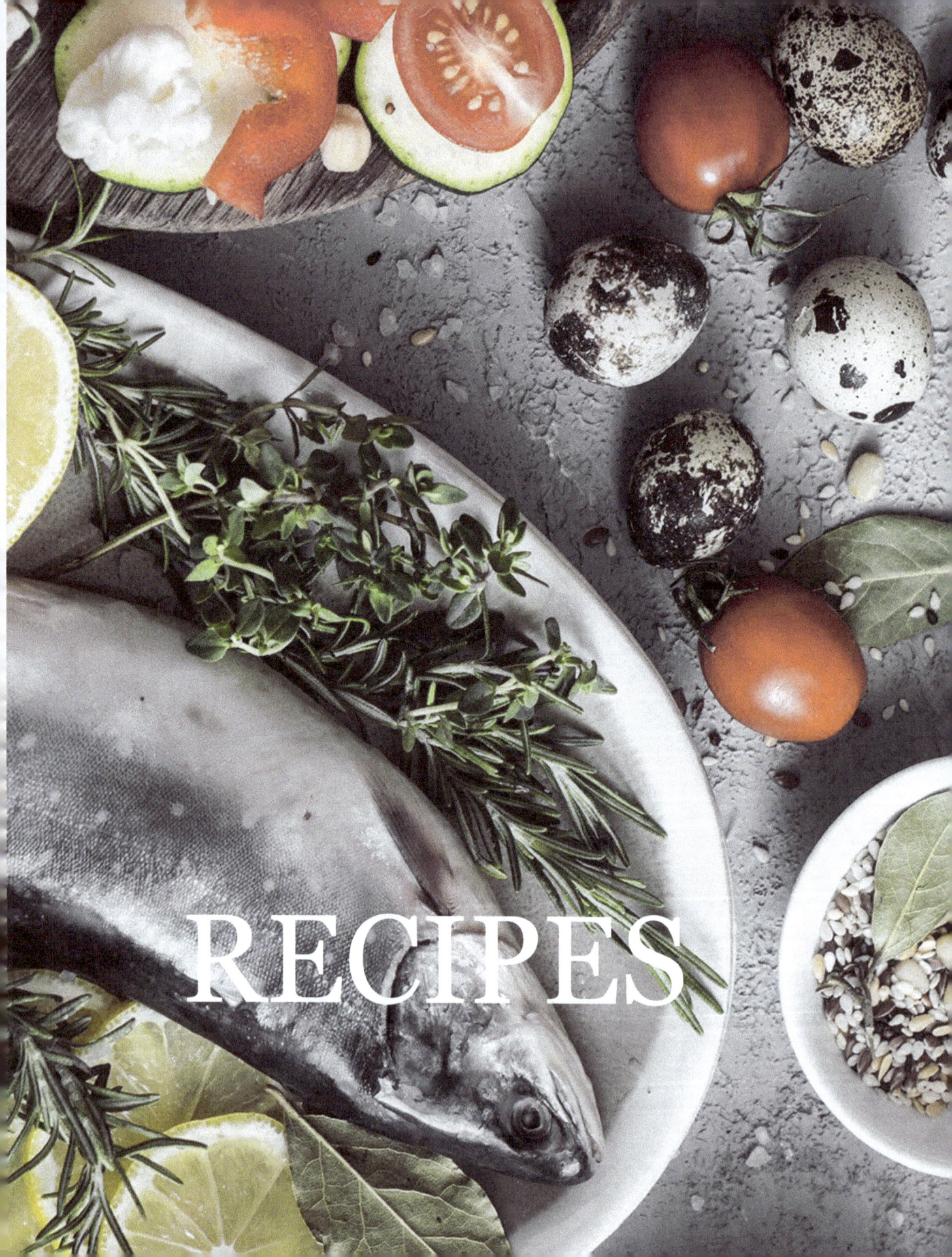

Salads

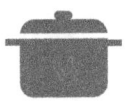

Pesto Chicken Pasta Salad

COOKING: 20 MIN　　　　　　　　　　　　　　SERVES: 2

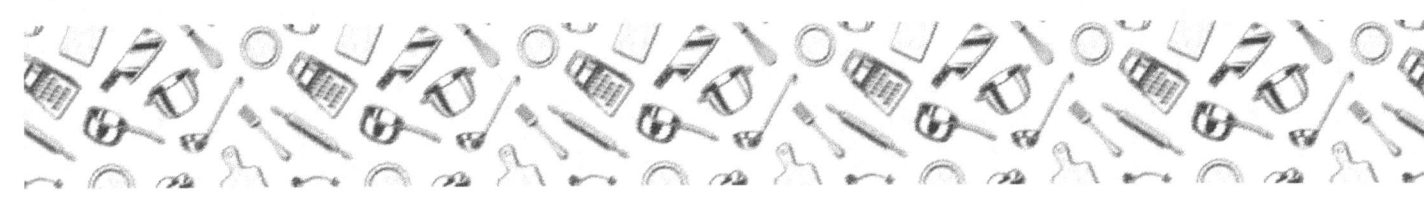

INGREDIENTS

Creamy Buttermilk Dressing:
1 large garlic clove, minced
1/3 cup mayonnaise
1/3 cup sour cream
1/3 cup buttermilk
3 tablespoons rice wine vinegar

Pasta Salad:
2 tablespoons salt
1-pound bow tie (farfalle) pasta
8 ounces trimmed asparagus, cut into 1-inch lengths
1-pound cooked chicken breast strips, pulled into bite-size pieces
8 ounces cherry tomatoes, halved and lightly salted
1 (14 ounce) can whole artichoke hearts, drained, cut into sixths
3 green onions, thinly sliced
1/2 cup pine nuts, toasted in a small skillet over low heat until golden
1/4 cup pesto (homemade or refrigerated prepared variety)

Nutritional Value: 250 calories per serving

DIRECTIONS

1. Mix dressing Ingredients in a small bowl; keep chilled until ready to toss with salad. (Store in clean jar with lid.)
2. Bring 1 gallon of water and 2 Tbs. of salt to boil in a large soup kettle. Add pasta and, using package times as a guide, boil, stirring frequently and adding asparagus the last 1 minute, until just tender. Drain thoroughly (do not rinse) and dump onto a large, lipped cookie sheet. Set aside to cool while preparing remaining salad Ingredients.
3. Place all salad Ingredients (except buttermilk dressing) in a large bowl or transfer to a gallon-size zippered bag. (Can be covered and refrigerated several hours at this point.) When ready to serve, add dressing; toss to coat and serve.

Salads

 **Asparagus and Artichoke Salad**

COOKING: 10 MIN   SERVES: 2

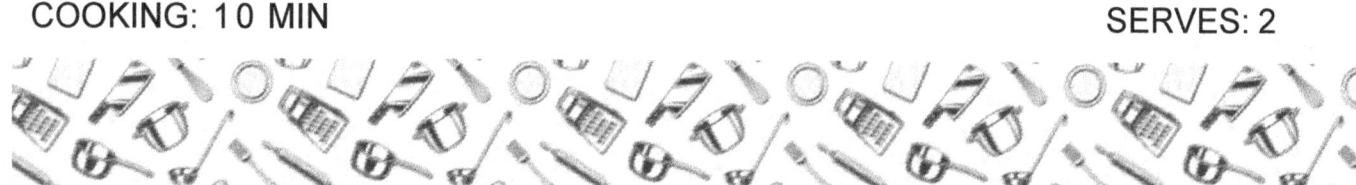

INGREDIENTS

6 slices bacon
10 asparagus spears, ends trimmed
1/2 (16 ounce) package rotini, elbow, or penne pasta
3 tablespoons low fat mayonnaise
3 tablespoons balsamic vinaigrette salad dressing
2 teaspoons lemon juice
1 teaspoon Worcestershire sauce
1 (6 ounce) jar marinated artichoke hearts, drained and coarsely chopped
1 cooked chicken breast, cubed
1/4 cup dried cranberries
1/4 cup toasted sliced almonds salt and pepper to taste

Nutritional Value: 150 calories per serving

DIRECTIONS

1. Place bacon in a large, deep skillet. Cook over medium high heat until evenly brown. Drain, crumble and set aside.
2. Meanwhile, bring a large pot of lightly salted water to a boil. Add asparagus and cook until tender, about 1 minute. Strain asparagus out of water and immediately plunge into a bowl filled with ice water; let sit in ice water until completely cold, then cut into 1 inch pieces. Next, add pasta to boiling water and cook for 8 to 10 minutes or until al dente; drain, rinse with cold water until chilled, then drain well.
3. Stir together mayonnaise, balsamic vinaigrette, lemon juice, and Worcestershire sauce in a large bowl. Fold in artichoke, chicken, cranberries, almonds, crumbled bacon, and asparagus. Season to taste with salt and pepper, then fold in cooked pasta. Refrigerate for at least 1 hour before serving.

Salads

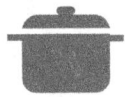

Chicken Spinach Salad

COOKING: 10 MIN

SERVES: 2

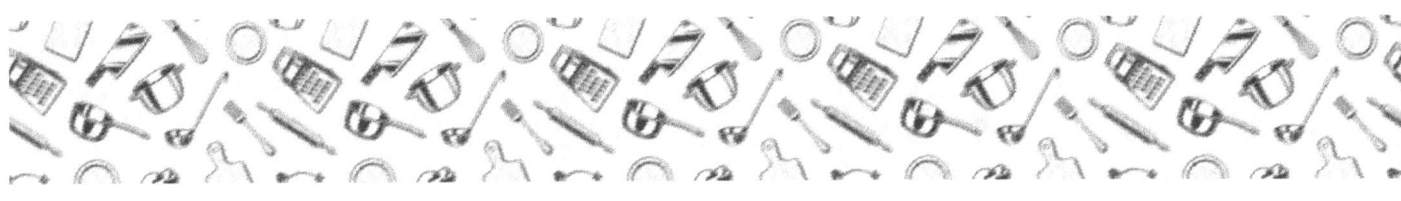

INGREDIENTS

1 (10 ounce) bag fresh spinach, rinsed and dried
4 cooked skinless, boneless chicken breast halves, sliced
1 zucchini, halved lengthwise and sliced
1 red bell pepper, chopped
1/2 cup black olives
3 ounces fontina cheese, shredded
1/2 cup fat-free roasted garlic salad dressing

Nutritional Value: 156 calories per serving

DIRECTIONS

1. Place equal portions of spinach onto four salad plates. Arrange chicken, zucchini, bell pepper, and black olives over spinach, and top with cheese. Drizzle dressing over salad.

Salads

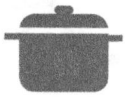

Wild Rice Salad

COOKING: 10 MIN

SERVES: 2

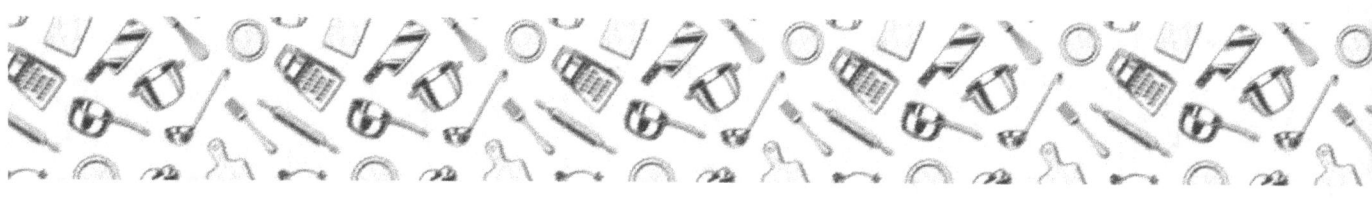

INGREDIENTS

2 (6 ounce) packages long grain and wild rice mix
2 avocados, peeled and chopped
1 (8 ounce) jar marinated whole mushrooms, undrained
1 (6.5 ounce) jar marinated artichoke hearts, undrained
2 medium tomatoes, diced
2 celery ribs, chopped
2 green onions, chopped
1/2 cup Italian salad dressing

Nutritional Value: 333 calories per serving

DIRECTIONS

1. Prepare the rice according to package Instructions. Cool; transfer to a large bowl. Add remaining Ingredients and toss to coat. Cover and refrigerate overnight.

Salads

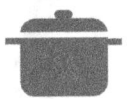

Tuna Salad

COOKING: 10 MIN   SERVES: 2

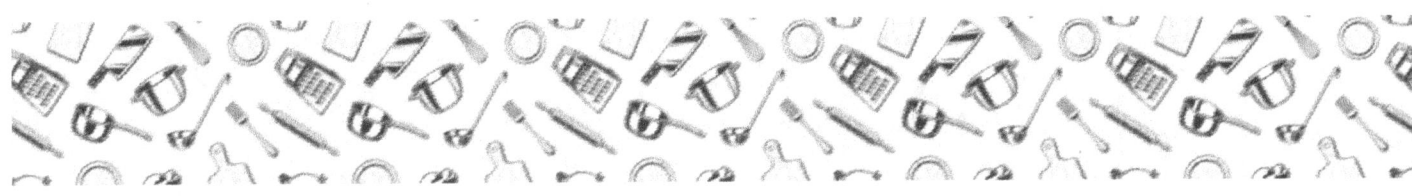

INGREDIENTS

2 (6 ounce) cans tuna, drained
1/2 head broccoli, finely chopped
1/2 head cauliflower, finely chopped
1/2 red onion, finely chopped
2 stalks celery, finely chopped
1 cup fat-free mayonnaise, or to taste
4 pita bread rounds

Nutritional Value: 250 calories per serving

DIRECTIONS

1. In a large bowl, toss together the tuna, broccoli, cauliflower, onion and celery. Stir in mayonnaise until the salad reaches your desired consistency. Serve on pita bread.

Salads

Mediterranean Olive Salad

COOKING: 10 MIN   SERVES: 2

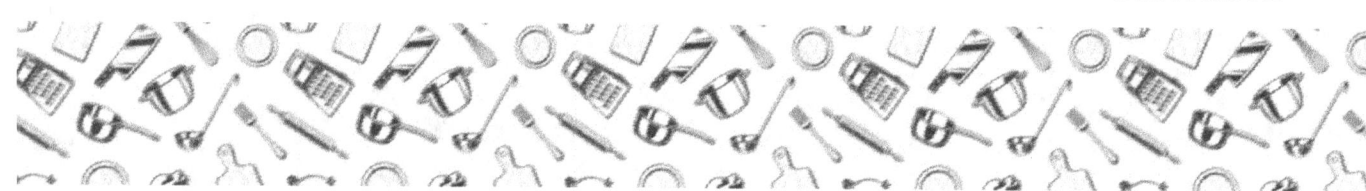

INGREDIENTS

1 (6 ounce) can black olives, drained
1 (5 ounce) jar pitted green olives, rinsed and drained
1 (6.5 ounce) jar marinated artichoke hearts, undrained
1 small red onion, chopped
1/4 cup red wine vinegar
1/2 cup olive oil
1 teaspoon dried minced garlic
1/2 teaspoon celery seed
1 teaspoon dried oregano
1 teaspoon dried basil
3/4 teaspoon black pepper

Nutritional Value: 155 calories per serving

DIRECTIONS

1. Place the black olives, green olives, artichoke hearts with their juice, and onion into a food processor. Pour in the vinegar and olive oil, and season with garlic, celery seed, oregano, basil and black pepper. Cover, and process until finely chopped. Use as a condiment on sandwiches, or a dip for crackers. Refrigerate leftovers.

Salads

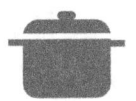 

Winter Vegetable Salad

COOKING: 20 MIN   SERVES: 2

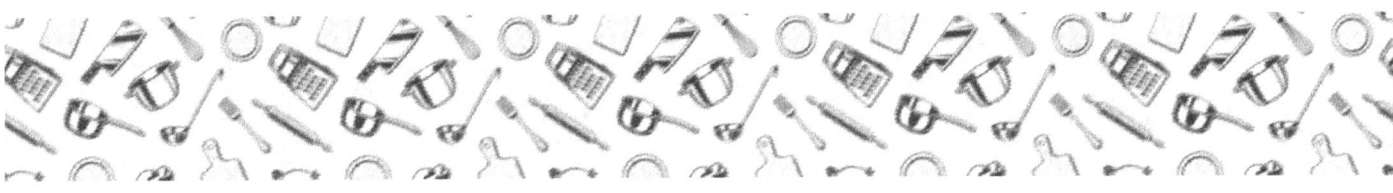

INGREDIENTS

1 (10 ounce) package mixed baby greens
1 red bell pepper, chopped
1 sweet potato, peeled and thinly sliced
2 stalks celery, chopped
1 jicama, peeled and thinly sliced
1 kohlrabi bulbs, peeled and diced
1 (14 ounce) can artichoke hearts in water, drained and halved
2 tablespoons olive oil
2 tablespoons fresh lemon juice
1/2 teaspoon oregano
1 teaspoon Greek seasoning salt and pepper to taste
3 pepperoncini peppers, minced
1/4 cup crumbled feta cheese

Nutritional Value: 147 calories per serving

DIRECTIONS

1. Layer the baby greens, bell pepper, sweet potato, celery, jicama, kohlrabi, and artichokes, in a salad bowl. Whisk together the olive oil, lemon juice, oregano, Greek seasoning, salt, and pepper in a small bowl. Drizzle over the salad, then sprinkle with pepperoncini and feta cheese to serve.

Salads

 Tomato, Cucumber and Onion Salad with Mint

COOKING: 10 MIN SERVES: 2

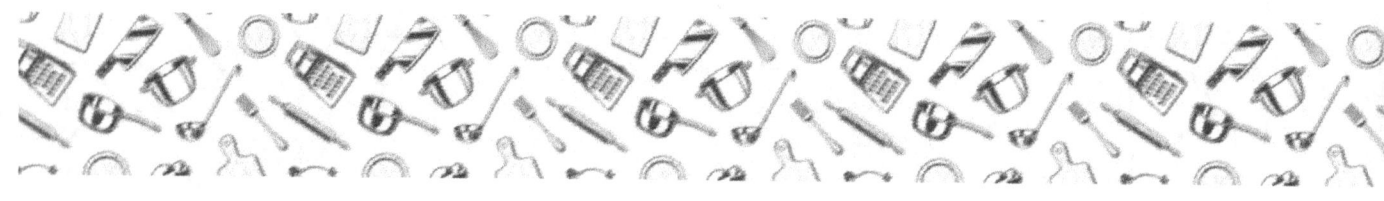

INGREDIENTS

2 large cucumbers - halved lengthwise, seeded and sliced
1/3 cup red wine vinegar
1 tablespoon white sugar
1 teaspoon salt
3 large tomatoes, seeded and coarsely chopped
2/3 cup coarsely chopped red onion
1/2 cup chopped fresh mint leaves
3 tablespoons olive oil salt and pepper to taste

Nutritional Value: 250 calories per serving

DIRECTIONS

1. In a large bowl, toss together the cucumbers, vinegar, sugar and salt. Let stand at room temperature for an hour, stirring occasionally.
2. Add tomatoes, onion, mint and oil to cucumbers and toss to blend. Season to taste with salt and pepper.

Salads

 Cabbage, Onion and Tomato Salad Greek Style

COOKING: 10 MIN   SERVES: 2

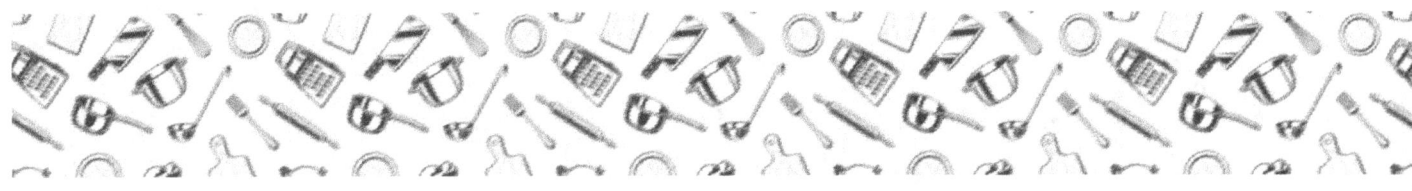

INGREDIENTS

2 cups shredded cabbage
4 large firm tomatoes, chopped
1 large onion, finely chopped
2 green chile peppers, seeded and minced
salt to taste
white sugar to taste
1 tablespoon roasted peanut powder
1 tablespoon clarified butter
1 teaspoon cumin seeds
1/2 cup chopped fresh cilantro

Nutritional Value: 125 calories per serving

DIRECTIONS

1. In a large bowl, toss together the cabbage, tomatoes, onion, chiles, salt, sugar and peanut powder until evenly combined.
2. In a small sauté pan, heat the clarified butter over medium heat. Add the cumin and stir until toasted. Remove from heat, pour over the salad mixture and gently mix together. Chill until serving and serve garnished with cilantro.

Salads

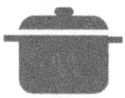 **Tuna Salad with Oranges and Pecans**

COOKING: 10 MIN   SERVES: 2

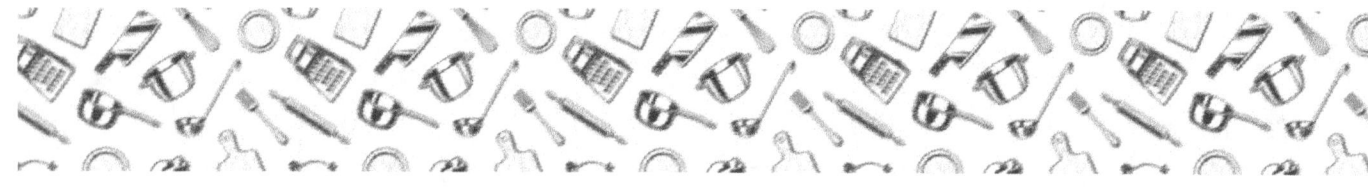

INGREDIENTS

1 (12 ounce) can water packed tuna, drained and flaked
1 tablespoon fat free sour cream
1/2 tablespoon mustard
1 1/2 tablespoons sweet pickle relish
2 tablespoons fresh orange juice
1/4 cup chopped pecans
garlic salt to taste onion powder to taste
ground black pepper to taste

Nutritional Value: 223 calories per serving

DIRECTIONS

1. Mix together the tuna, sour cream, mustard, relish, orange juice, pecans, garlic salt, onion powder, and black pepper. Cover and refrigerate until ready to use.

Salads

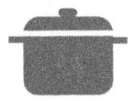

Asparagus Salad Italian Way

COOKING: 10 MIN   SERVES: 2

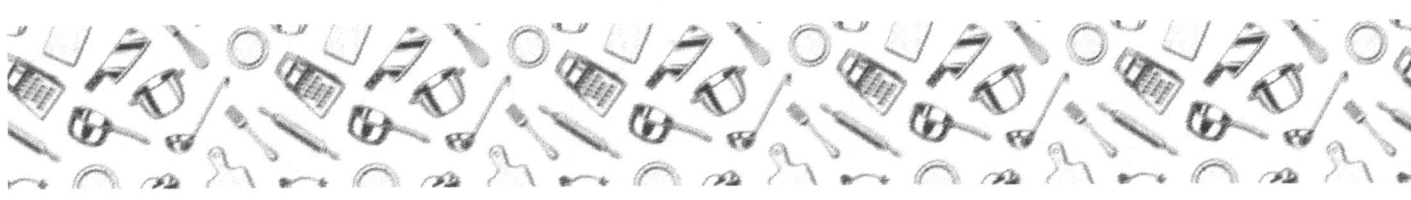

INGREDIENTS

1/2 cup Blue Cheese Italian Vinaigrette Dressing
1 1/4 pounds fresh asparagus, trimmed
1/4 cup pine nuts
3 roasted red peppers, packed in water, cut into 1/4-inch pieces
1/4 cup chopped fresh parsley

Nutritional Value: 124 calories per serving

DIRECTIONS

1. Bring a large pot of water to a boil. Cook asparagus for 1 minute. Drain. Rinse and cool under cold water. Pat asparagus dry with paper towels. Preheat oven to 350 degrees F. Toast pine nuts for 5 -7 minutes. Cool.
2. Arrange asparagus on a platter, top with peppers and parsley. Pour Marzetti Italian Blue Cheese Crumble Dressing overall. Sprinkle with toasted pine nuts. Serve.

Salads

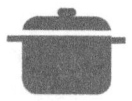 **Salad with Spinach and Cranberries**

COOKING: 10 MIN   SERVES: 2

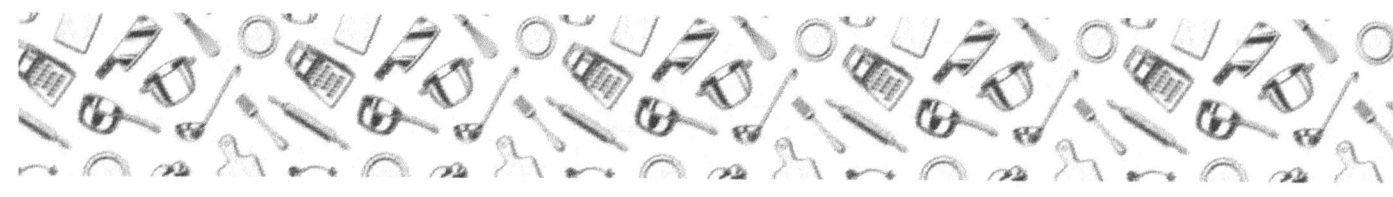

INGREDIENTS

1 (6 ounce) package fresh baby spinach
1/2 cup chopped pecans, toasted
1/2 cup dried cranberries
1/3 cup olive or vegetable oil
3 tablespoons sugar
2 tablespoons red wine or balsamic vinegar
1 tablespoon sour cream
1/2 teaspoon Dijon mustard

Nutritional Value: 139 calories per serving

DIRECTIONS

1. In a bowl, combine the spinach, pecans and cranberries. In a jar with a tight-fitting lid, combine the remaining Ingredients; shake well. Drizzle over salad and toss to coat; serve immediately.

Salads

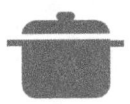

Spinach, Peaches and Pecan Salad

COOKING: 10 MIN   SERVES: 2

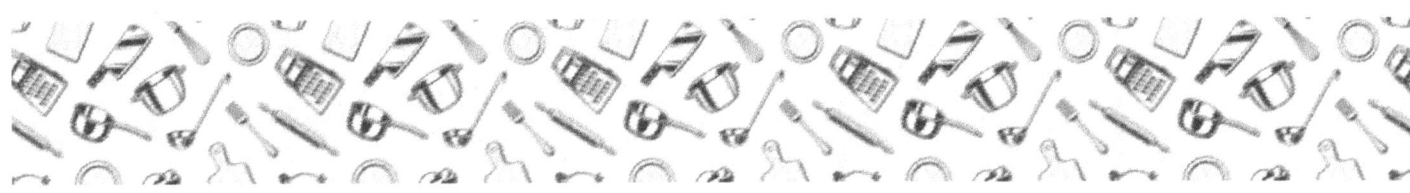

INGREDIENTS

3/4 cup pecans
2 ripe peaches
4 cups baby spinach, rinsed and dried
1/4 cup poppyseed salad dressing

Nutritional Value: 405 calories per serving

DIRECTIONS

1. Preheat oven to 350 degrees F (175 degrees C). Arrange pecans on a single layer on a baking sheet and roast in preheated oven for 7-10 minutes, until they just begin to darken. Remove from oven and set aside.
2. Peel peaches (if desired) and slice into bite-sized segments. Combine peaches, spinach and pecans in a large bowl. Toss with dressing until evenly coated, adding a little additional dressing, if necessary.

Salads

 **Cold Rice Salad**

COOKING: 10 MIN   SERVES: 2

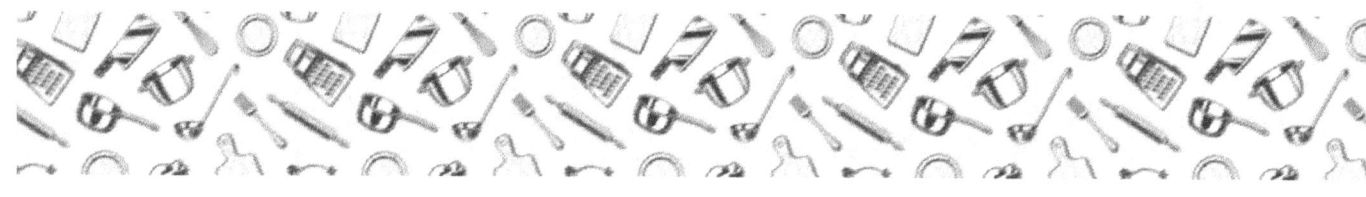

INGREDIENTS

1 (6.9 ounce) package chicken-flavored rice and vermicelli mix
1 teaspoon vegetable oil
12 stuffed green olives, sliced
4 green onions, thinly sliced
1/2 green pepper, chopped
2 (6.5 ounce) jars marinated artichoke hearts, drained, liquid reserved
1/3 cup mayonnaise
1/2 teaspoon curry powder

Nutritional Value: 385 calories per serving

DIRECTIONS

1. Prepare rice mix according to package Instructions, except substitute 1 teaspoon oil for butter called for. Cool. Add olives, green onions and green pepper; toss to mix. Cut the artichokes into quarters and add to rice mixture; set aside. In a small bowl, combine mayonnaise, curry powder and reserved marinade, blend well. Pour over rice mixture; toss to mix. Cover and chill for at least 2 hours.

.

Salads

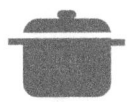

Spinach Salad with Mustard

COOKING: 10 MIN   SERVES: 2

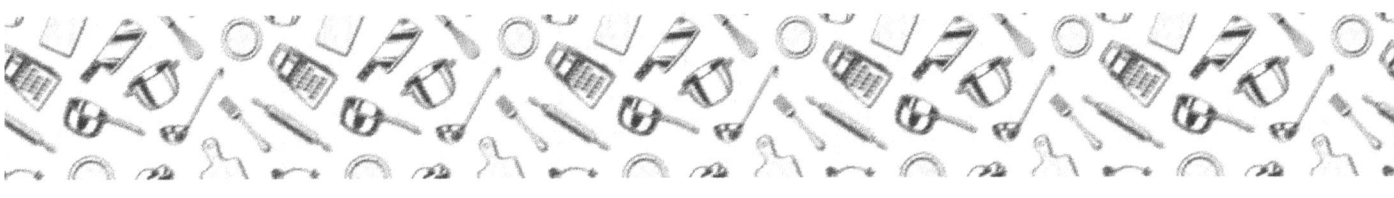

INGREDIENTS

1 (10 ounce) bag baby spinach leaves
4 hard-cooked eggs, peeled and sliced
1 cup sliced mushrooms
4 strips crisply cooked bacon, crumbled
10 ounces Swiss cheese, shredded
1/2 cup toasted sliced almonds
1 tablespoon olive oil
1 large shallot, minced
1 teaspoon garlic, minced
1/3 cup white wine vinegar
1/3 cup Dijon mustard
1/3 cup honey
2 strips crisply cooked bacon, crumbled
salt and pepper to taste

Nutritional Value: 318 calories per serving

DIRECTIONS

1. Place spinach into a large serving bowl, top with hard-cooked eggs, mushrooms, 4 crumbled strips of bacon, Swiss cheese, and almonds.
2. Heat olive oil in a small skillet over medium heat. Stir in shallots and garlic, and cook until softened and translucent, about 2 minutes.
3. Whisk in the vinegar, Dijon mustard, honey, and 2 crumbled strips of bacon; season to taste with salt and pepper, then cook until hot.
4. Pour hot dressing over spinach and toss to coat.

Salads

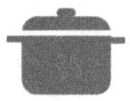 **Spinach Salad with Pork Meat**

COOKING: 10 MIN   SERVES: 2

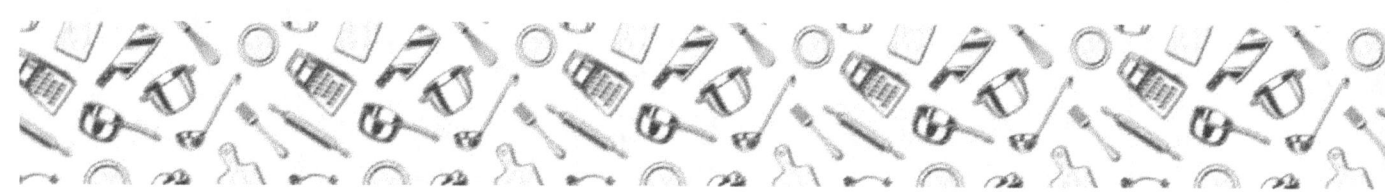

INGREDIENTS

10 ounces fresh spinach, washed, stems removed
1 (15.5 ounce) can black-eyed peas, rinsed and drained
1/3 cup Italian or low-fat Italian dressing
1/4 cup sliced green onions
1/2 cup sliced fresh mushrooms
1/4 cup sliced celery
1 (2 ounce) jar sliced pimentos, drained
2 tablespoons sliced ripe olives
2 garlic cloves, minced
1 tablespoon olive oil
1/2-pound pork tenderloin, cut into thin strips

DIRECTIONS

1. Line four plates with spinach leaves; set aside. In a bowl, combine peas, mushrooms, Italian dressing, green onions, celery, pimientos, and olives; set aside. In a medium skillet, sauté garlic in oil for 30 seconds. Add pork and stir-fry for 2 to 3 minutes or until no pink remains. Remove from the heat; add vegetable mixture and mix well. Divide among spinach-lined plates. Serve immediately.

Nutritional Value: 417 calories per serving

Salads

Linguine and Shrimp Salad

COOKING: 10 MIN SERVES: 2

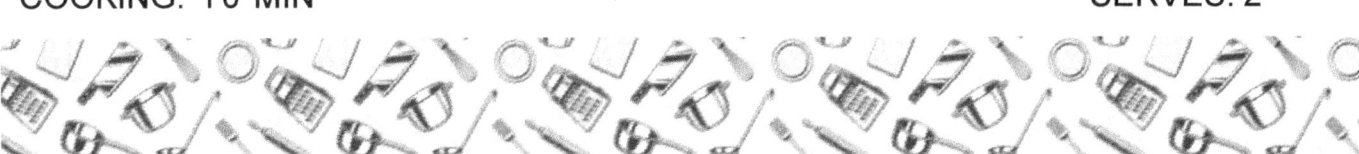

INGREDIENTS

8 ounces uncooked linguine pasta, broken in half
1-pound cooked medium shrimp, peeled and deveined
3 cups fresh broccoli florets
1 (14 ounce) can water packed artichoke hearts, drained and chopped
1/2-pound fresh mushrooms, sliced
12 cherry tomatoes, halved
3/4 cup shredded carrots
1/2 cup sliced green onions
1/3 cup olive oil or canola oil
1/3 cup reduced-sodium soy sauce
1 tablespoon lemon juice
1 garlic clove, minced
1/2 teaspoon hot pepper sauce
2 tablespoons sesame seeds, toasted

Nutritional Value: 250 calories per serving

DIRECTIONS

1. Cook linguine according to package Instructions; drain and rinse in cold water. Place in a bowl; add the shrimp, broccoli, artichokes, mushrooms, tomatoes, carrots and onions.
2. In a jar with a tight-fitting lid, combine the oil, soy sauce, lemon juice, garlic and hot pepper sauce; shake well. Pour over salad and toss to coat. Cover and refrigerate for at least 1 hour. Just before serving, sprinkle with sesame seeds.

Salads

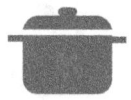 Artichoke and White Bean Salad

COOKING: 10 MIN SERVES: 2

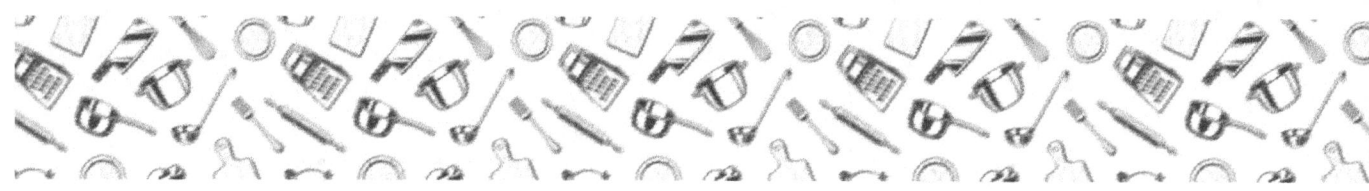

INGREDIENTS

3 cups white beans, drained
1/2 (14 ounce) can artichoke hearts, drained and quartered
2/3 cup diced green bell pepper
1/3 cup chopped black olives
1/4 cup chopped red onion
1/4 cup chopped fresh parsley
1/4 ounce chopped fresh mint leaves
3/4 teaspoon dried basil
1/3 cup olive oil
1/4 cup red wine vinegar

Nutritional Value: 265 calories per serving

DIRECTIONS

1. In a large bowl, combine beans, artichoke hearts, bell peppers, olives, onion, parsley, mint, and basil.
2. In a jar or small bowl, combine oil and vinegar; shake together or mix well. Pour oil and vinegar over the salad and toss to coat.
3. Cover and chill in refrigerator for several hours or overnight, stirring occasionally, to let flavors blend.

Salads

Spinach Salad with Goat Cheese

COOKING: 10 MIN   SERVES: 2

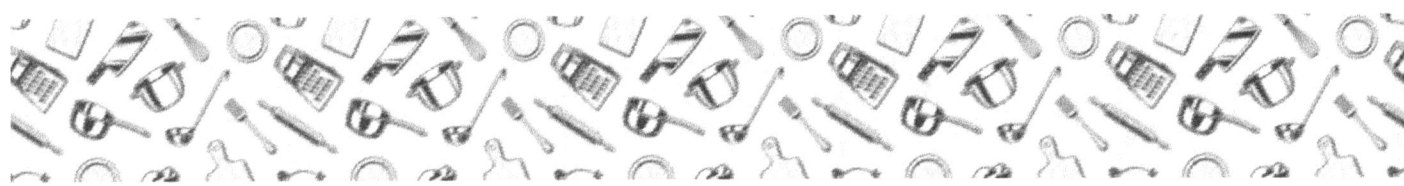

INGREDIENTS

8 cups baby spinach, rinsed and dried
1 tablespoon butter
1 clove garlic, crushed
1/4 cup plain breadcrumbs
6 ounces goat cheese, sliced
8 tablespoons balsamic vinegar
8 tablespoons olive oil

Nutritional Value: 208 calories per serving

DIRECTIONS

1. Arrange the spinach on four plates.
2. In a skillet, melt butter over medium heat, and add crushed garlic. Cook and stir until slightly golden. Stir in breadcrumbs. Drop the goal cheese slices into the breadcrumbs a few at a time and turn to coat in the breadcrumb mixture.
3. Place a slice or two of goat cheese on each serving of spinach and drizzle the salads with olive oil and balsamic vinegar.

Salads

Artichoke Salad vol.2

COOKING: 10 MIN   SERVES: 2

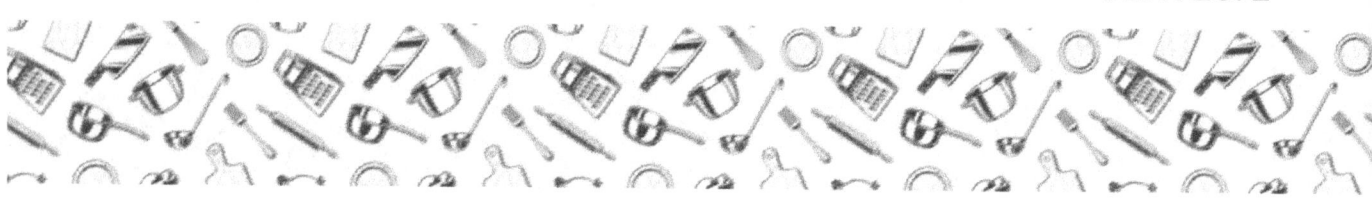

INGREDIENTS

4 cups mixed salad greens
1/2 red onion, sliced
1 (14 ounce) can artichoke hearts in water, drained
1/2 cup vegetable oil
1/2 cup red wine vinegar
1 teaspoon seasoned salt
1 teaspoon ground black pepper
1 teaspoon garlic powder
3 tablespoons grated Parmesan cheese

Nutritional Value: 147 calories per serving

DIRECTIONS

1. In a large bowl, combine the mixed greens, onion, and artichoke hearts.

2. In a medium-size mixing bowl, whisk together the oil, vinegar, seasoned salt, pepper, and garlic.

3. Pour enough dressing over salad to coat and toss well. Sprinkle with grated cheese and serve.

Salads

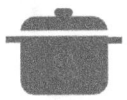

Seven Spinach Salad

COOKING: 20 MIN   SERVES: 2

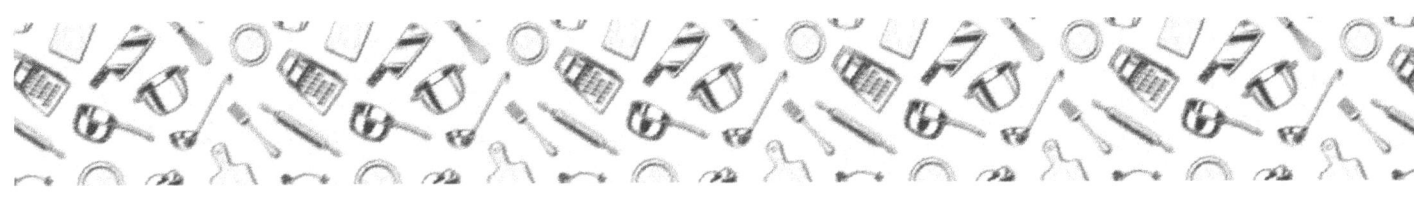

INGREDIENTS

1 (6 ounce) package baby spinach leaves
1/3 cup cubed Cheddar cheese
1 Fuji apple - peeled, cored and diced
1/3 cup finely chopped red onion
1/4 cup sweetened dried cranberries
1/3 cup blanched slivered almonds
3 tablespoons poppy seed salad dressing

Nutritional Value: 250 calories per serving

DIRECTIONS

1. In a large salad bowl, combine the spinach, Cheddar cheese, apple, red onion, cranberries and slivered almonds. Toss with poppy seed dressing just before serving.

Salads

 **Spinach, Berries and Curry Salad**

COOKING: 10 MIN   SERVES: 2

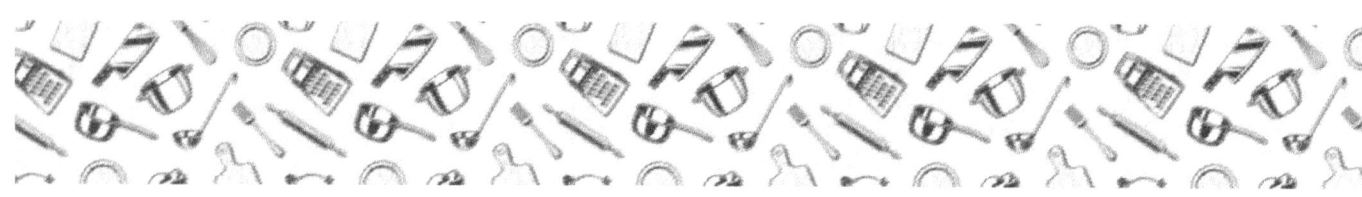

INGREDIENTS

6 cups fresh spinach, torn into bite-size pieces
1 cup thickly sliced strawberries
1 cup blueberries, trimmed
1 small red onion, thinly sliced
1/2 cup chopped pecans
Non-Fat Curry Dressing:
2 tablespoons balsamic vinegar
2 tablespoons rice vinegar
4 teaspoons honey
1 teaspoon curry powder
2 teaspoons Dijon mustard
1 pinch Salt and pepper to taste

Nutritional Value: 365 calories per serving

DIRECTIONS

1. Wash and dry spinach. Whip together dressing Ingredients. Add to spinach and toss lightly. Add berries, onion and pecans. Toss lightly and serve.

Salads

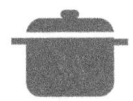 **Spinach Salad with Raspberries**

COOKING: 10 MIN   SERVES: 2

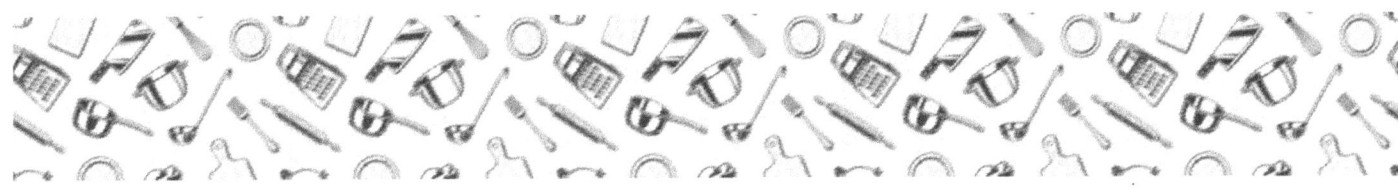

INGREDIENTS

3 tablespoons vegetable oil
2 tablespoons raspberry vinegar
2 tablespoons raspberry jam
1/8 teaspoon pepper
8 cups torn fresh spinach
2 cups fresh raspberries, divided
4 tablespoons slivered almonds, toasted and divided
1/2 cup thinly sliced onion
3 kiwifruits, peeled and sliced
1 cup seasoned salad croutons

Nutritional Value: 258 calories per serving

DIRECTIONS

1. In a jar with a tight-fitting lid, combine the oil, vinegar, jam and pepper; shake well. In a large salad bowl, gently combine spinach, 1 cup of raspberries, 2 tablespoons almonds and onion. Top with kiwi, croutons and remaining berries and almonds. Drizzle with dressing; serve immediately.

Salads

 **Rice Salad with Artichokes**

COOKING: 10 MIN   SERVES: 2

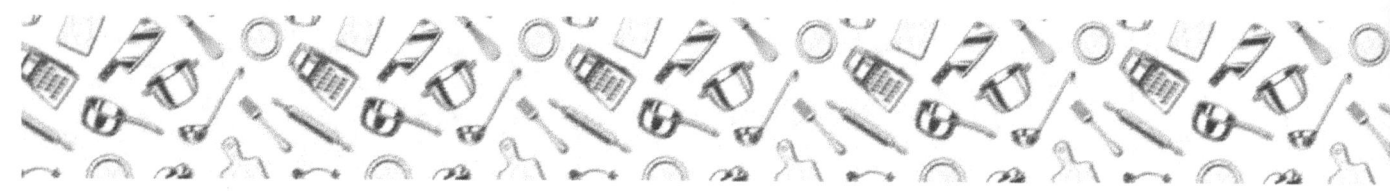

INGREDIENTS

1 (6.9 ounce) package chicken-flavored rice and vermicelli mix
2 (6.5 ounce) jars marinated artichoke hearts
3 cups cooked long-grain rice
3 cups chopped green onions
3/4 cup mayonnaise
1/2 teaspoon curry powder

Nutritional Value: 369 calories per serving

DIRECTIONS

1. Prepare rice mix according to package Instructions; cool. Drain artichokes, reserving marinade. Chop artichokes; place in a large bowl. Add prepared rice, long grain rice and onions. In a small bowl, combine mayonnaise, curry powder and reserved marinade. Pour over rice mixture and toss to coat. Cover and refrigerate until serving.

Salads

Ranch Salad

COOKING: 10 MIN   SERVES: 2

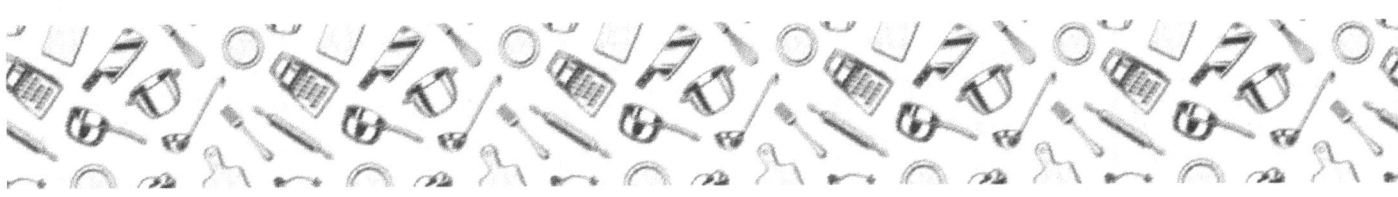

INGREDIENTS

4 cups baby spinach, rinsed and dried
1/2 cup cucumber
1 cup broccoli florets
1/2 cup feta cheese, crumbled
1/4 red onion, chopped
2 small, cooked chicken breasts, cut into small pieces bacon bits
1/2 cup ranch dressing

Nutritional Value: 150 calories per serving

DIRECTIONS

1. Toss together spinach, cucumber, broccoli, feta, onion, chicken, and bacon in a large bowl. Pour dressing over salad, and gently toss again.

Salads

 **Strawberry Salad with Sunflowers**

COOKING: 10 MIN   SERVES: 2

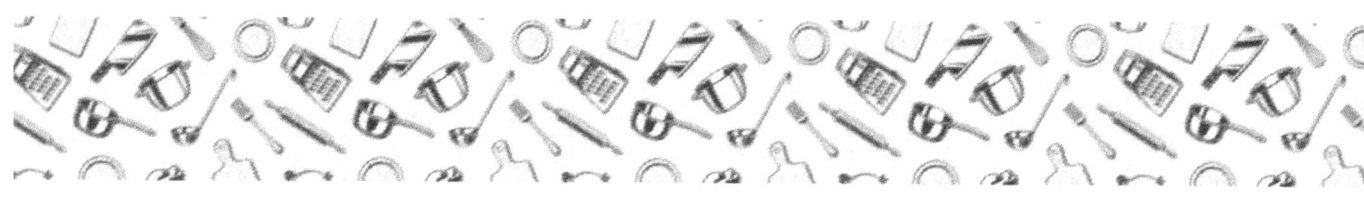

INGREDIENTS

2 cups sliced fresh strawberries
1 medium apple, diced
1 cup seedless green grapes, halved
1/2 cup thinly sliced celery
1/4 cup raisins
1/2 cup strawberry yogurt
2 tablespoons sunflower seeds
Lettuce Leaves

Nutritional Value: 250 calories per serving

DIRECTIONS

1. In a large bowl, combine strawberries, apple, grapes, celery and raisins. Stir in the yogurt. Cover and refrigerate for at least 1 hour. Add sunflower seeds and toss; serve on lettuce leaves if desired.

Salads

Anna's Salad

COOKING: 10 MIN   SERVES: 2

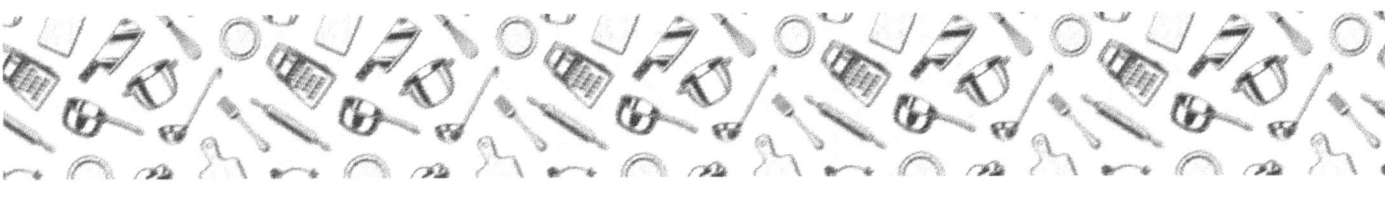

INGREDIENTS

2/3 cup vegetable oil
1/4 cup red wine vinegar
2 teaspoons lemon juice
2 teaspoons soy sauce 1 teaspoon sugar
1 teaspoon dry mustard
1/2 teaspoon curry powder
1/2 teaspoon salt
1/2 teaspoon seasoned pepper
1/4 teaspoon garlic powder
1 (10 ounce) package fresh spinach, torn into bite-size pieces
5 bacon strips, cooked and crumbled
2 hard-cooked eggs, sliced

Nutritional Value: 123 calories per serving

DIRECTIONS

1. Combine first 10 Ingredients in a jar; cover tightly and shake until well mixed; set aside. Place spinach in a large salad bowl. Just before serving, pour dressing over spinach and toss gently. Garnish with crumbled bacon and egg slices.

Salads

Tomato, Onion and Corn Salad

COOKING: 10 MIN   SERVES: 2

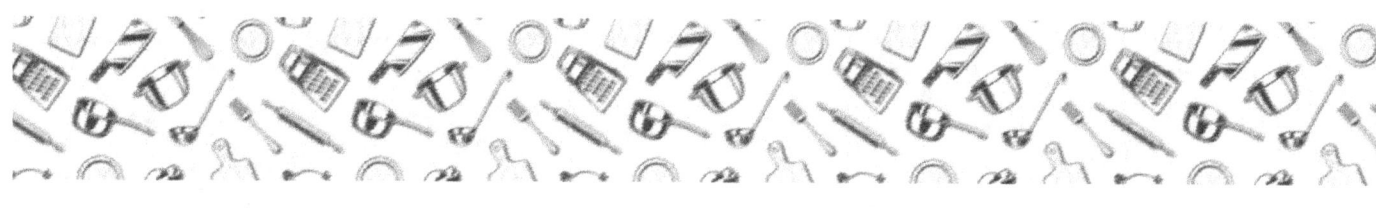

INGREDIENTS

3 (11 ounce) cans whole kernel corn
2 large tomatoes, diced
1 large sweet onion, cut into thin strips
4 green onions, chopped
1 bunch cilantro leaves, minced into tiny strips
2 limes, juiced
1/3 cup rice vinegar kosher salt to taste

Nutritional Value: 258 calories per serving

DIRECTIONS

1. In a large bowl, combine corn, tomatoes, sweet onion, green onion, and cilantro. Squeeze lime juice over mixture, and mix in. Stir in rice vinegar to taste; the amount you use will depend on the sweetness of the corn, and the acidity of the lime. Season with kosher salt.
2. Cover, and chill for 45 minutes to an hour. Stir before serving.

Salads

Pesto Chicken Pasta Salad

COOKING: 20 MIN SERVES: 2

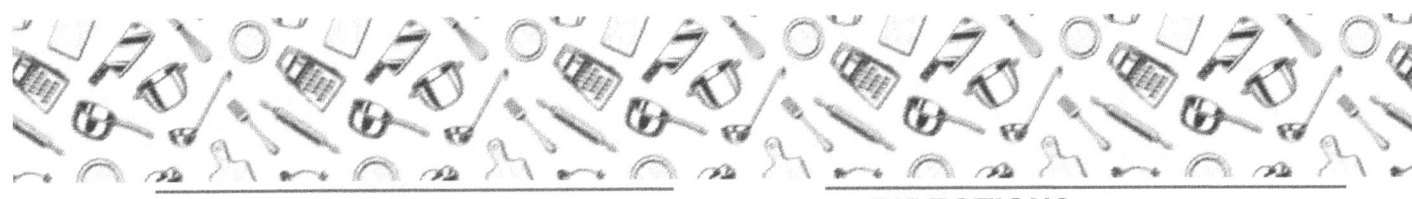

INGREDIENTS

Creamy Buttermilk Dressing:
1 large garlic clove, minced
1/3 cup mayonnaise
1/3 cup sour cream
1/3 cup buttermilk
3 tablespoons rice wine vinegar
Pasta Salad:
2 tablespoons salt
1-pound bow tie (farfalle) pasta
8 ounces trimmed asparagus, cut into 1-inch lengths
1-pound cooked chicken breast strips, pulled into bite-size pieces
8 ounces cherry tomatoes, halved and lightly salted
1 (14 ounce) can whole artichoke hearts, drained, cut into sixths
3 green onions, thinly sliced
1/2 cup pine nuts, toasted in a small skillet over low heat until golden
1/4 cup pesto (homemade or refrigerated prepared variety)
Nutritional Value: 250 calories per serving

DIRECTIONS

1. Mix dressing Ingredients in a small bowl; keep chilled until ready to toss with salad. (Store in clean jar with lid.)
2. Bring 1 gallon of water and 2 Tbs. of salt to boil in a large soup kettle. Add pasta and, using package times as a guide, boil, stirring frequently and adding asparagus the last 1 minute, until just tender. Drain thoroughly (do not rinse) and dump onto a large, lipped cookie sheet. Set aside to cool while preparing remaining salad Ingredients.
3. Place all salad Ingredients (except buttermilk dressing) in a large bowl or transfer to a gallon-size zippered bag. (Can be covered and refrigerated several hours at this point.) When ready to serve, add dressing; toss to coat and serve.

Salads

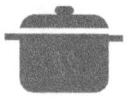 

French Salad

COOKING: 10 MIN   SERVES: 2

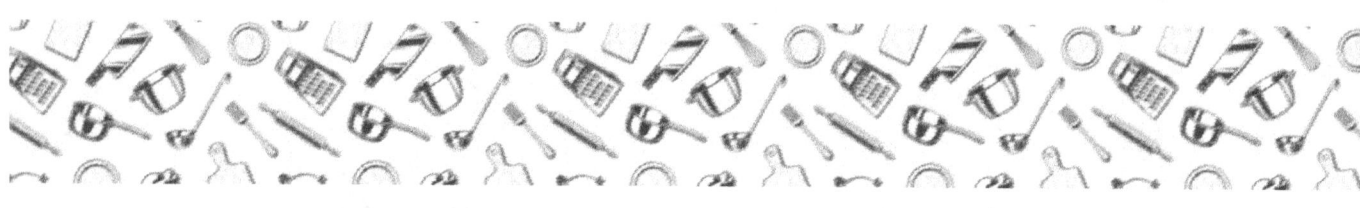

INGREDIENTS

1-pound fresh asparagus
3/4-pound cooked shrimp - peeled and deveined
1/3 cup mayonnaise
1 tablespoon lemon juice
6 artichoke hearts, drained
1 cup French dressing
2 hard-cooked eggs, chopped
6 sprigs fresh parsley

Nutritional Value: 250 calories per serving

DIRECTIONS

1. Cook the asparagus in boiling salted water until tender. Remove and cool under cold water. Reserve six stalks and cut remaining asparagus into 1-inch pieces.
2. Cook and clean shrimp. Again, reserve the best six and dice the remainder. In a bowl, combine shrimp and asparagus, mix gently with mayonnaise and lemon juice.
3. In a separate bowl, marinate the artichoke hearts in 1 cup French dressing.
4. Place shrimp and asparagus in an attractive shallow bowl. Garnish with sieved egg and arrange reserved asparagus on top to resemble the spokes of a wheel.
5. Drain the artichoke bottoms and garnish each with a dollop of mayonnaise, 1 whole shrimp and 1 parsley sprig. Arrange them around the salad.

Salads

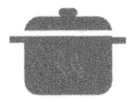

Red Onion and Orange Salad

COOKING: 20 MIN

SERVES: 2

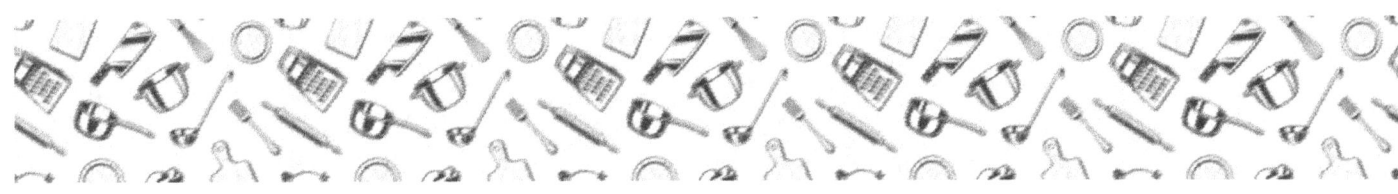

INGREDIENTS

4 cups torn romaine
2 cups medium navel oranges, peeled and sectioned
1 small red onion, sliced and separated into rings
1/4 cup olive oil
3 tablespoons red wine vinegar
1 teaspoon sugar
1/4 teaspoon salt
1/8 teaspoon pepper

DIRECTIONS

1. On a serving platter, arrange the romaine, oranges and onion. In a jar with a tight-fitting lid, combine the remaining Ingredients; shake well. Drizzle over salad; serve immediately

Salads

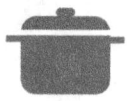 **Watermelon and Avocado Salad**

COOKING: 10 MIN   SERVES: 2

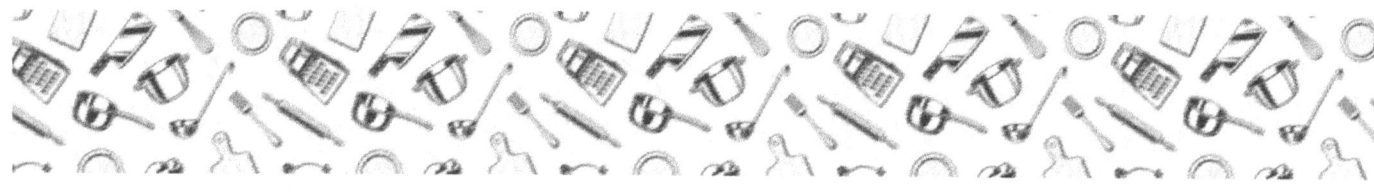

INGREDIENTS

2 large avocados - peeled, pitted and diced
4 cups cubed watermelon
4 cups fresh spinach leaves
1 cup balsamic vinaigrette salad dressing

Nutritional Value: 250 calories per serving

DIRECTIONS

1. In a salad bowl, toss together the avocado, watermelon cubes and spinach. Stir in salad dressing just before serving.

Salads

Asparagus and Strawberries Salad

COOKING: 10 MIN   SERVES: 2

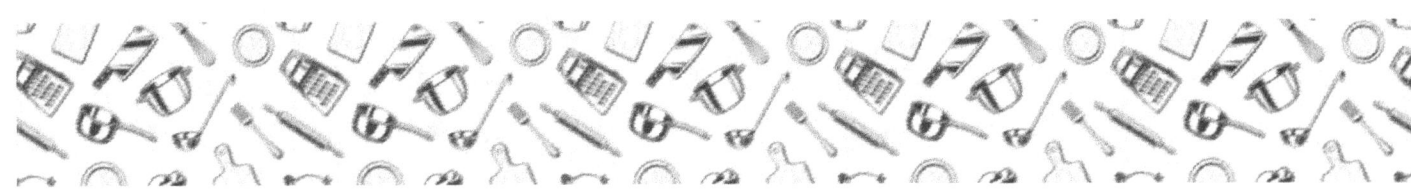

INGREDIENTS

1/4 cup lemon juice
2 tablespoons vegetable oil
2 tablespoons honey
2 cups fresh asparagus, cut into 1-inch pieces
2 cups sliced fresh strawberries

Nutritional Value: 321 calories per serving

DIRECTIONS

1. In a small bowl, combine lemon juice, oil and honey; mix well. Cook asparagus in a small amount of water until crisp-tender, about 3-4 minutes; drain and cool. Arrange asparagus and strawberries on individual plates, drizzle with dressing.

Salads

Tomato and Basil Salad

COOKING: 10 MIN

SERVES: 2

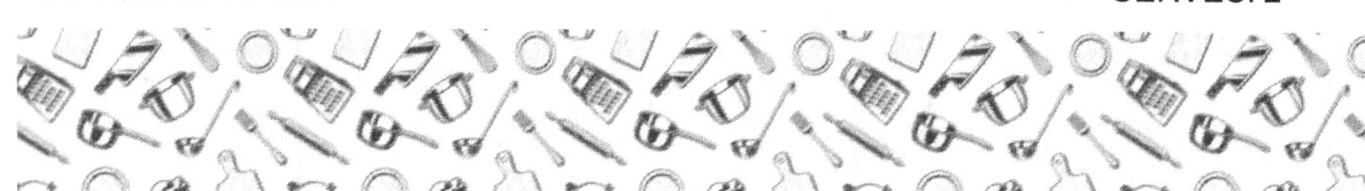

INGREDIENTS

2 pints cherry tomatoes, halved salt, to taste
1/4 cup mayonnaise
1/4 cup sour cream
2 tablespoons rice wine vinegar
1 garlic clove, minced
3 cups fresh corn kernels
1/4 cup torn basil leaves
1 small red onion, quartered and thinly sliced
1/2 cup raisins
Salt
Pepper

Nutritional Value: 250 calories per serving

DIRECTIONS

1. Salt tomatoes in a bowl and set aside. Whisk together mayonnaise, sour cream, vinegar and garlic; set aside. Add corn, basil, onion and raisins to tomatoes. Season with salt and pepper and toss with dressing.

Salads

Daiquiri Salad

COOKING: 10 MIN SERVES: 2

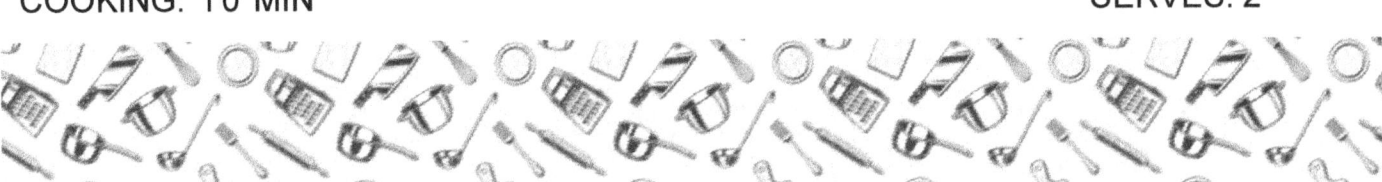

INGREDIENTS

1/4 cup lime juice
1/4 cup honey
1/4 teaspoon poppy seeds
1/4 teaspoon Dijon mustard
1/4 cup vegetable oil
1 cup sliced almonds
1/4 teaspoon salt
1/4 cup white sugar
1 bag baby spinach, rinsed and dried
2 pints sliced fresh strawberries
1 cup toasted flaked coconut
1/2 red onion, sliced

Nutritional Value: 253 calories per serving

DIRECTIONS

1. Combine the lime juice, honey, poppy seeds, and mustard in a small bowl; slowly whisk in the oil.
2. Combine the almonds, salt, and sugar in a large skillet. Stir constantly over medium-low heat until almonds are light golden brown, about 5 minutes. Remove nuts from the skillet to cool.
3. Toss the spinach, strawberries, coconut, onions, and cooled almonds in a large bowl. Top with prepared dressing and toss to coat.

Salads

Feta Artichoke Salad

COOKING: 10 MIN   SERVES: 2

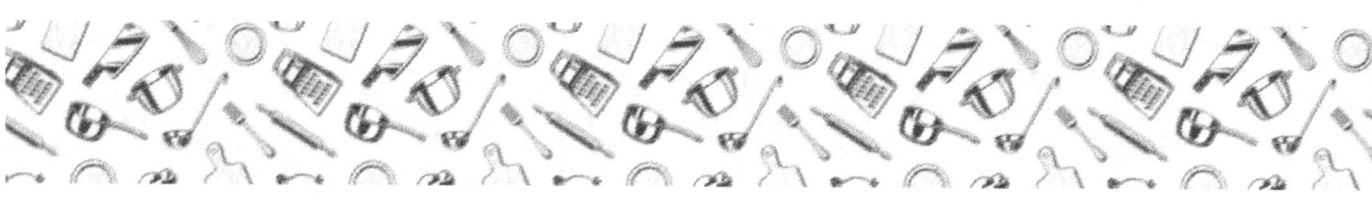

INGREDIENTS

1 tablespoon olive oil
1 (10 ounce) package spinach - rinsed, stemmed, and dried
1 red onion, thinly sliced
1 (8 ounce) jar marinated artichoke hearts
1 cup crumbled feta cheese

Nutritional Value: 146 calories per serving

DIRECTIONS

1. Preheat oven to 300 degrees F (150 degrees C).
2. Drizzle olive oil on a rimmed baking sheet. Spread spinach leaves in a thick layer covering the baking sheet. Arrange onions and artichokes over the spinach and drizzle the marinade from the jar over the entire salad. Sprinkle with the cheese (and sausage, if you wish). Bake for about 10 minutes, or until the spinach is wilted but NOT crispy.

Salads

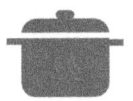

Peanut Apple Salad

COOKING: 10 MIN   SERVES: 2

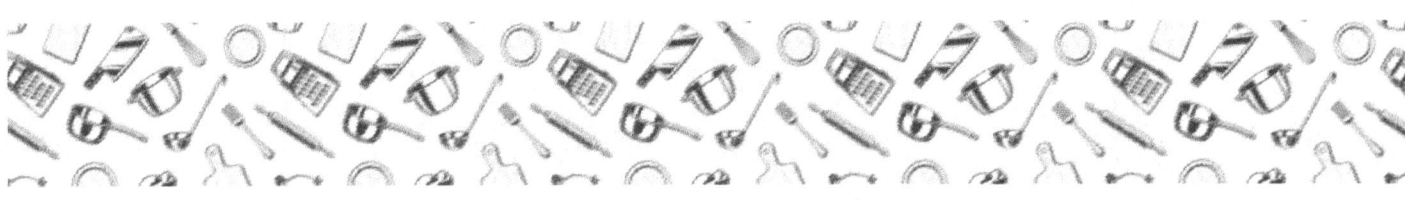

INGREDIENTS

2 (6 ounce) packages fresh baby spinach
1 medium apple, chopped
1/4 cup raisins
2 tablespoons chopped peanuts
2 tablespoons olive oil
1 tablespoon sugar
1 tablespoon cider vinegar
1 tablespoon chutney
3/4 teaspoon curry powder 1/4 teaspoon salt

Nutritional Value: 280 calories per serving

DIRECTIONS

1. In a large bowl, combine the spinach, apple, raisins and peanuts. In a jar with a tight-fitting lid, combine the remaining Ingredients; shake well. Drizzle over salad and toss to coat.

Salads

Onion and Strawberry Salad

COOKING: 10 MIN SERVES: 2

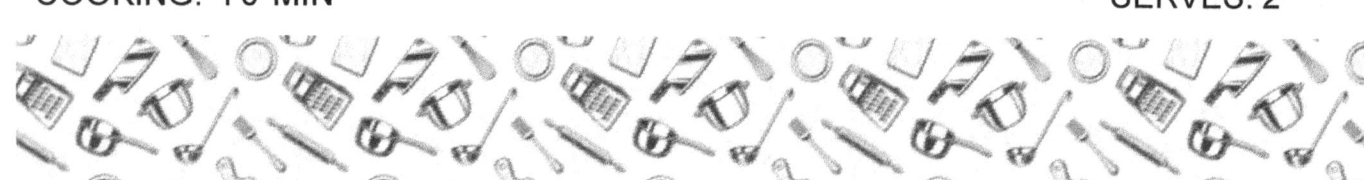

INGREDIENTS

1/4 cup mayonnaise
1/4 cup sour cream
2 tablespoons red wine vinegar
1/3 cup white sugar
1/4 cup milk
2 tablespoons poppy seeds
1-pint fresh strawberries, sliced
1 head red leaf lettuce, rinsed and torn
1 red onion, thinly sliced

Nutritional Value: 302 calories per serving

DIRECTIONS

1. In a small bowl, mix together the mayonnaise, sour cream, red wine vinegar, sugar, milk and poppy seeds. Set aside.
2. Divide the lettuce into 6 individual salad bowls. Sprinkle strawberries over the lettuce, and garnish with onion slices. Pour dressing over salads just before serving.

Salads

 Chicken Salad vol.2

COOKING: 10 MIN

SERVES: 2

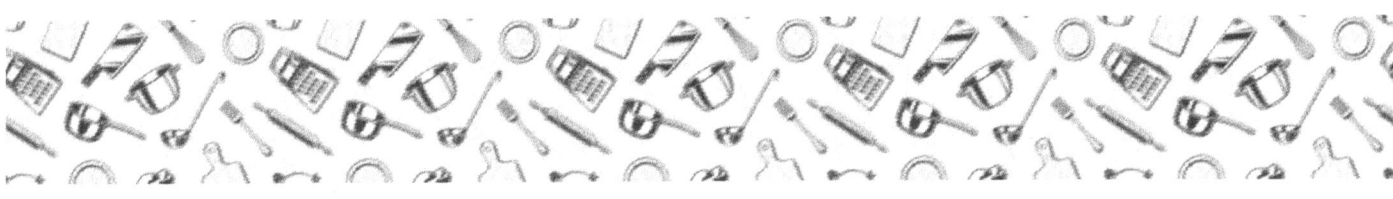

INGREDIENTS

1 can cream of chicken soup
2 c. cooked chicken
3/4 c. mayonnaise
1 tsp. lemon juice
1 c. chopped celery
1/2 sm. onion, diced
1/4 c. chopped pimento
1/2 tsp. pecan or almond, chopped
3 hardboiled eggs, chopped
2 c. crushed potato chips

Nutritional Value: 361 calories per serving

DIRECTIONS

1. Mix together all Ingredients except potato chips. Top with crushed chips. Bake at 400 degrees for 20 minutes until bubbly.

Salads

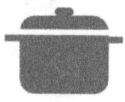 **Spinach and Pepper Jelly Dressing Salad**

COOKING: 10 MIN   SERVES: 2

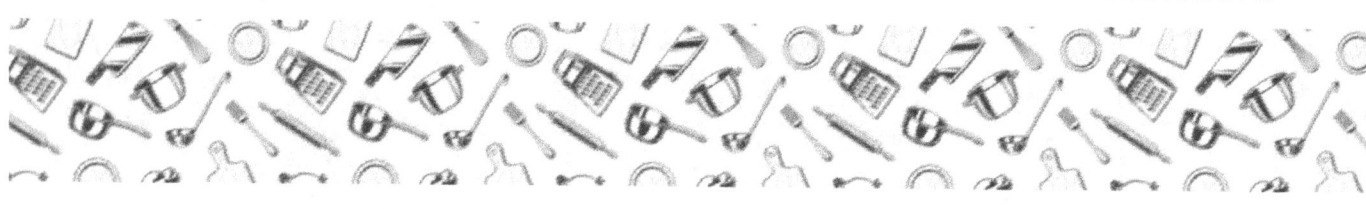

INGREDIENTS

3 tablespoons mild pepper jelly
2 tablespoons olive oil
1/8 teaspoon salt
1/8 teaspoon Dijon mustard
2 cups baby spinach leaves
2 ounces goat cheese, sliced
2 tablespoons chopped walnuts

Nutritional Value: 358 calories per serving

DIRECTIONS

1. In a small bowl, whisk together the pepper jelly, olive oil, salt and mustard to make the dressing. Heat in the microwave for 30 seconds. Let cool.
2. Place the spinach in a large bowl and toss with the dressing. Divide between two serving bowls. Top each one with slices of goat cheese and sprinkle with walnuts.

Salads

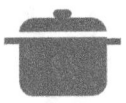 Feta, Couscous and Asparagus Salad

COOKING: 10 MIN   SERVES: 2

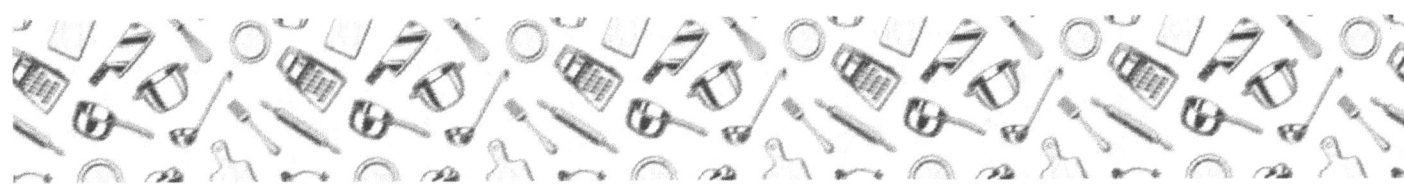

INGREDIENTS

2 cups couscous
1 bunch fresh asparagus, trimmed and cut into 2-inch pieces
8 ounces grape tomatoes, halved
6 ounces feta cheese, crumbled
3 tablespoons balsamic vinegar
2 tablespoons extra-virgin olive oil
Pepper

Nutritional Value: 430 calories per serving

DIRECTIONS

1. Cook couscous according to package instructions. Put aside and allow to cool slightly.
2. Meanwhile, place asparagus in a steamer over 1 inch of boiling water, and cover. Cook until tender but still firm, about 2 to 6 minutes. Drain and cool.
3. Toss the asparagus, tomatoes, and feta with couscous. Add the olive oil, balsamic vinegar, and black pepper and toss to incorporate.

Salads

Pork and Walnuts Salad

COOKING: 10 MIN SERVES: 2

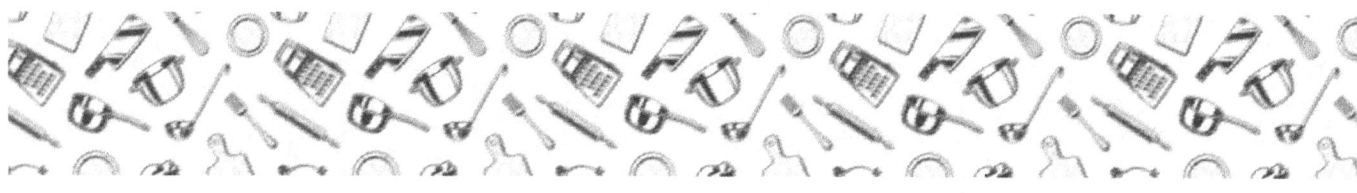

INGREDIENTS

1 tablespoon olive oil
1-pound pork tenderloin, cut into 1-inch cubes
1 tablespoon chopped fresh parsley
1 (10 ounce) bag fresh spinach leaves
1 Asian pear, cored and sliced 1/4 cup chopped walnuts
1/2 cup balsamic vinaigrette salad dressing, or to taste

Nutritional Value: 458 calories per serving

DIRECTIONS

1. Heat the oil in a large skillet over medium-high heat. Add the pork and parsley; cook and stir until pork is browned on the outside and cooked through. Remove from the heat and set aside.
2. Make a bed of spinach on individual serving plates or on a large platter. Arrange slices of pear over the spinach. Top with the cooked pork and sprinkle with walnuts. Drizzle the balsamic vinaigrette over the whole salad.

Salads

Pomegranate Salad

COOKING: 10 MIN

SERVES: 2

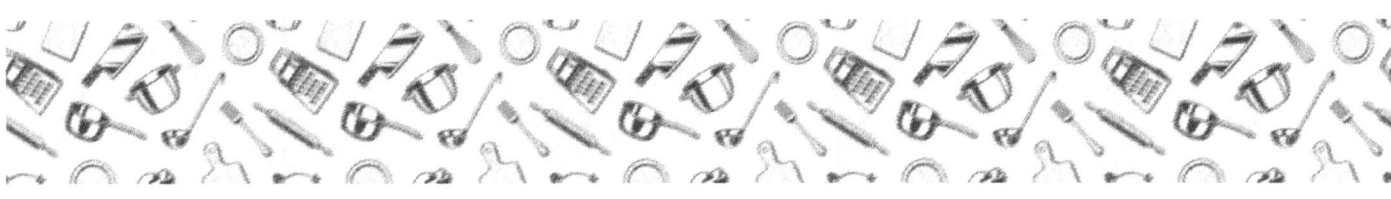

INGREDIENTS

1 (10 ounce) bag baby spinach leaves, rinsed and drained
1/4 red onion, sliced very thin
1/2 cup walnut pieces
1/2 cup crumbled feta
1/4 cup alfalfa sprouts (optional)
1 pomegranate, peeled and seeds separated
4 tablespoons balsamic vinaigrette

Nutritional Value: 250 calories per serving

DIRECTIONS

1. Place spinach in a salad bowl. Top with red onion, walnuts, feta, and sprouts. Sprinkle pomegranate seeds over the top, and drizzle with vinaigrette.

Salads

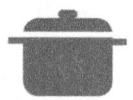 **Broccoli and Strawberry Salad**

COOKING: 10 MIN   SERVES: 2

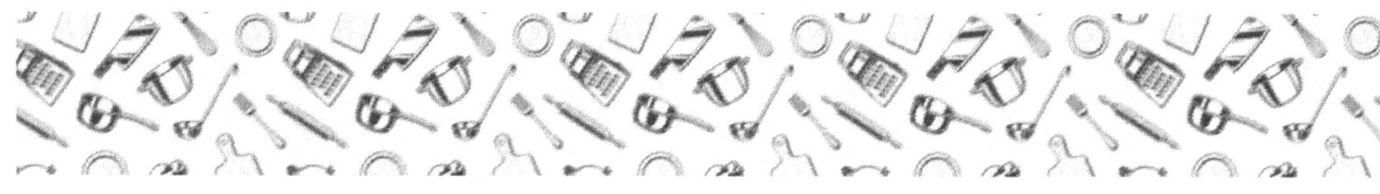

INGREDIENTS

1 1/2 cups chopped fresh broccoli
1 1/2 cups chopped fresh cauliflower
1/2 cup shredded carrot
5 fresh strawberries, sliced
1/4 cup slivered almonds
1/4 cup raspberry vinaigrette

Nutritional Value: 158 calories per serving

DIRECTIONS

1. Combine the broccoli, cauliflower, carrot, strawberries, almonds, and vinaigrette in a large bowl; toss to coat evenly. Serve immediately.

Salads

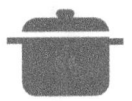 

Blackberry Salad

COOKING: 10 MIN   SERVES: 2

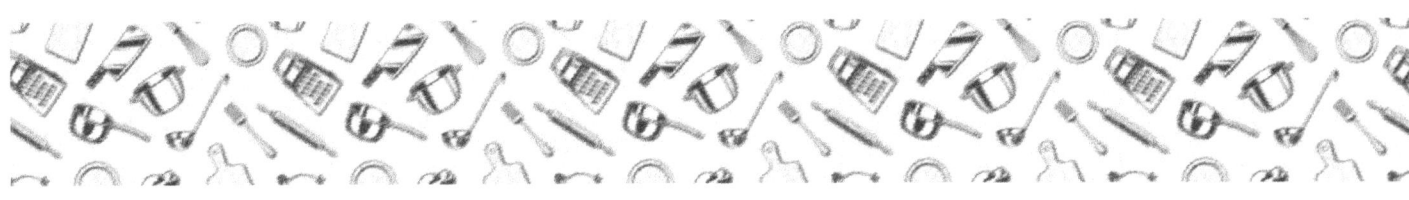

INGREDIENTS

3 cups baby spinach, rinsed and dried
1-pint fresh blackberries
6 ounces crumbled feta cheese
1-pint cherry tomatoes, halved
1 green onion, sliced
1/4 cup finely chopped walnuts (optional)
1/2 cup edible flowers (optional)

Nutritional Value: 258 calories per serving

DIRECTIONS

1. In a large bowl, toss together baby spinach, blackberries, feta cheese, cherry tomatoes, green onion, and walnuts. Garnish with edible flowers.

Salads

Strawberry Ginger Salad

COOKING: 10 MIN

SERVES: 2

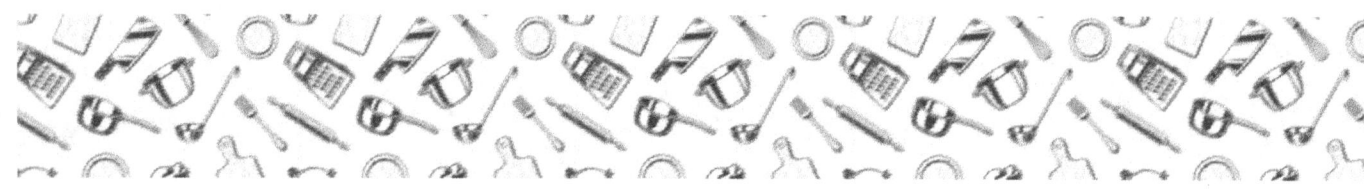

INGREDIENTS

2 teaspoons corn oil
1 skinless, boneless chicken breast half - cut into bite-size pieces
1/2 teaspoon garlic powder
1 1/2 tablespoons mayonnaise
1/2 lime, juiced
1/2 teaspoon ground ginger
2 teaspoons milk
2 cups fresh spinach, stems removed
4 fresh strawberries, sliced
1 1/2 tablespoons slivered almonds
Pepper

Nutritional Value: 158 calories per serving

DIRECTIONS

1. Heat oil in a skillet over medium heat. Place chicken in skillet, season with garlic powder and cook 10 minutes on each side or until juices run clear. Set aside.
2. In a bowl, mix mayonnaise, lime juice, ginger and milk.
3. Arrange spinach on serving dishes. Top with chicken and strawberries, sprinkle with almonds and drizzle with dressing. Season with pepper to serve.

Salads

Chicken and Almond Salad

COOKING: 10 MIN SERVES: 2

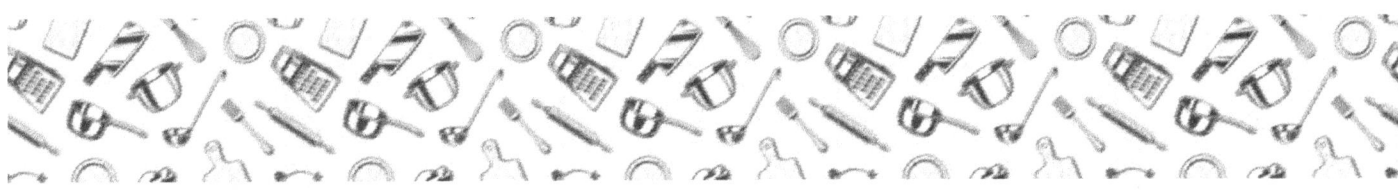

INGREDIENTS

4 cups cubed, cooked chicken
2 tablespoons fresh lemon juice
1 cup creamy salad dressing, e.g. Miracle Whip в„ў
1 teaspoon salt
1 cup pineapple tidbits, drained
1 cup halved green grapes
1 cup blanched slivered almonds, toasted
1/2 cup chopped water chestnuts
1/4 cup shredded lettuce

2.
3. **Nutritional Value**: 410 calories per serving

DIRECTIONS

1. In a large bowl, toss the chicken with the lemon juice. Cover and chill for 2 hours.
2. Mix the salad dressing, salt, pineapple, grapes, almonds, water chestnuts and lettuce into the chicken until evenly combined. Chill until serving.

Salads

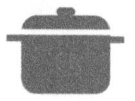

Asparagus Salad

COOKING: 10 MIN

SERVES: 2

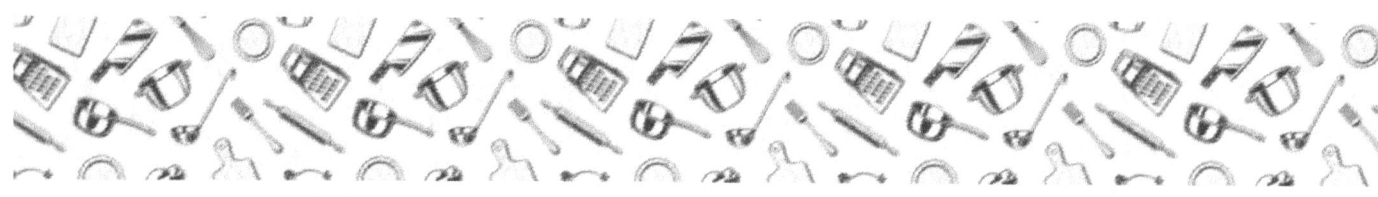

INGREDIENTS

1 1/4 pounds fresh asparagus, cut into 2-inch pieces
1 (4 ounce) jar diced pimientos, drained
1/3 cup sliced green onions
1/2 cup olive or vegetable oil
1/4 cup cider or white wine vinegar
1 teaspoon Dijon mustard
1 teaspoon Worcestershire sauce
1/2 teaspoon dried basil
1/2 teaspoon salt
1/4 teaspoon pepper
1/4 teaspoon dried thyme

Nutritional Value: 230 calories per serving

DIRECTIONS

1. In a saucepan, cook the asparagus in a small amount of water for 5 minutes or until crisp-tender. Rinse with cold water; drain well.
2. Place in a bowl; add pimientos and onions. In a small bowl, whisk oil, vinegar, mustard, Worcestershire sauce, basil, salt, pepper and thyme; pour over asparagus mixture and toss to coat. Cover and refrigerate for at least 2 hours. Serve with a slotted spoon.

Salads

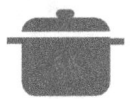

Romaine Salad

COOKING: 10 MIN

SERVES: 2

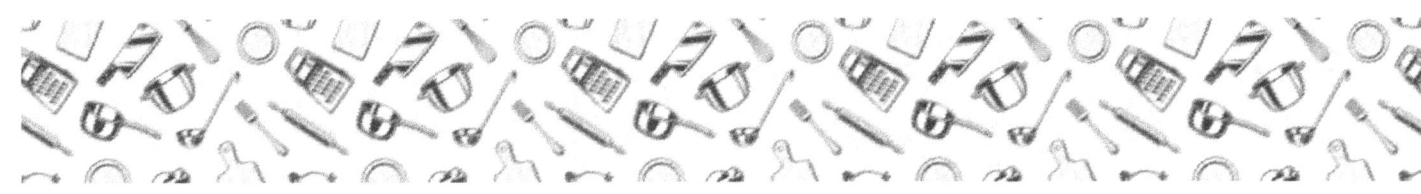

INGREDIENTS

1 head romaine lettuce - rinsed, dried, and chopped
2 bunches fresh spinach - chopped, washed and dried
1-pint fresh strawberries, sliced
1 Bermuda onion, sliced
1/2 cup mayonnaise
2 tablespoons white wine vinegar
1/3 cup raw honey
1/4 cup milk
2 tablespoons poppy seeds

Nutritional Value: 312 calories per serving

DIRECTIONS

1. In a large salad bowl, combine the romaine, spinach, strawberries and sliced onion.
2. In a jar with a tight-fitting lid, combine the mayonnaise, vinegar, sugar, milk and poppy seeds. Shake well and pour the dressing over salad. Toss until evenly coated.

Salads

Fruit Salad with Spinach

COOKING: 10 MIN

SERVES: 2

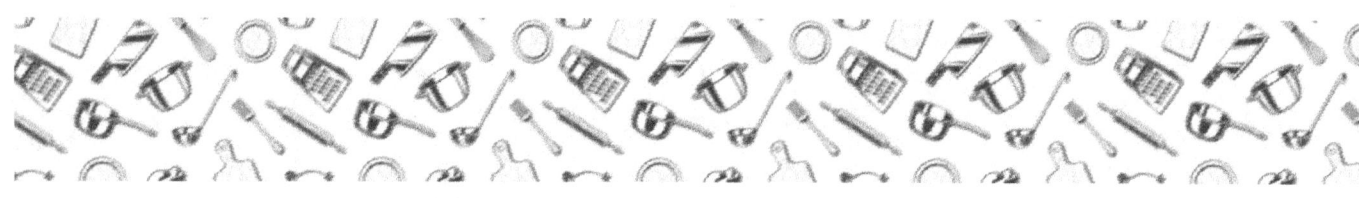

INGREDIENTS

1 (11 ounce) can mandarin oranges
1/4 cup olive or vegetable oil
3 tablespoons raspberry jam or spreadable fruit
1 tablespoon red wine vinegar
1 (10 ounce) package fresh spinach, torn
1 red apple, chopped
1 cup chopped pecans, toasted

Nutritional Value: 321 calories per serving

DIRECTIONS

1. Drain oranges, reserving 1/2 cup juice. In a jar with tight-fitting lid, combine oil, jam, vinegar and reserved juice; shake well. In a large salad bowl, toss oranges, spinach, apple and pecans. Serve with the dressing.

Salads

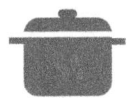

Cashew and Pecan Salad

COOKING: 10 MIN   SERVES: 2

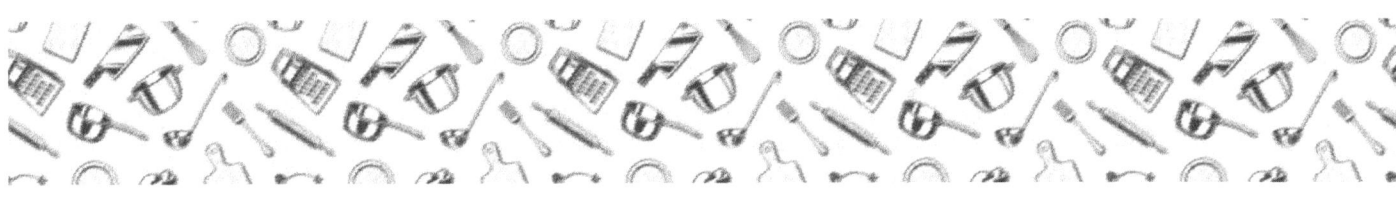

INGREDIENTS

1 cup honey
2 tablespoons ground cinnamon
2 1/2 cups cashews
2 cups frozen raspberries, thawed
1/2 cup red wine vinegar
1/2 cup extra virgin olive oil
3 chopped hearts of romaine
1 (10 ounce) bag fresh baby spinach
3 pears, cored and diced
1/2 cup dried cherries
1 cup feta cheese

Nutritional Value: 258 calories per serving

DIRECTIONS

1. Line a baking sheet with aluminum foil. Place the honey and cinnamon into a saucepan. Melt the sugar over medium heat without stirring. Add the cashews, and stir until well coated, then spread out onto the prepared baking sheet to cool to room temperature.
2. Puree the raspberries, vinegar, and olive oil until smooth; set aside. Toss together the romaine, spinach, pears, cherries, and feta cheese in a large bowl. Toss with half of the raspberry dressing, and sprinkle with candied cashews. Serve with remaining dressing on the side.

Salads

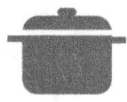 **Onion, Tomato and Cucumber Salad**

COOKING: 10 MIN   SERVES: 2

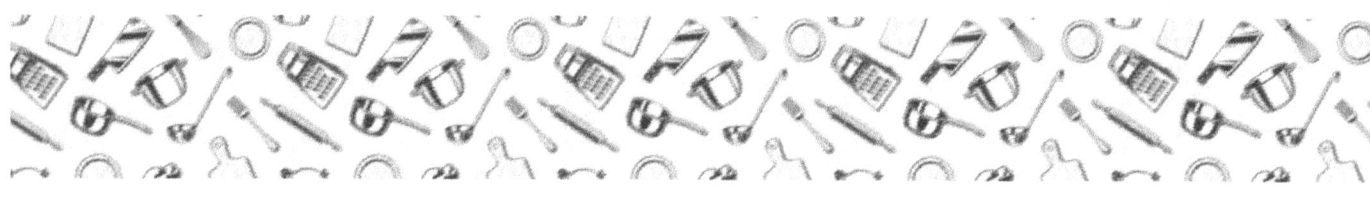

INGREDIENTS

4 tomatoes, cut into 8 wedges
2 large cucumbers, peeled and sliced
1 large red onion, chopped
1/4 cup chopped fresh cilantro juice of 1 fresh lime
Salt

Nutritional Value: 211 calories per serving

DIRECTIONS

1. Mix the tomatoes, cucumbers, red onion, cilantro, and lime juice together in a bowl. Season with salt to serve.

Salads

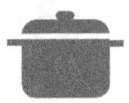

Blue Cheese and Strawberry Salad

COOKING: 10 MIN   SERVES: 2

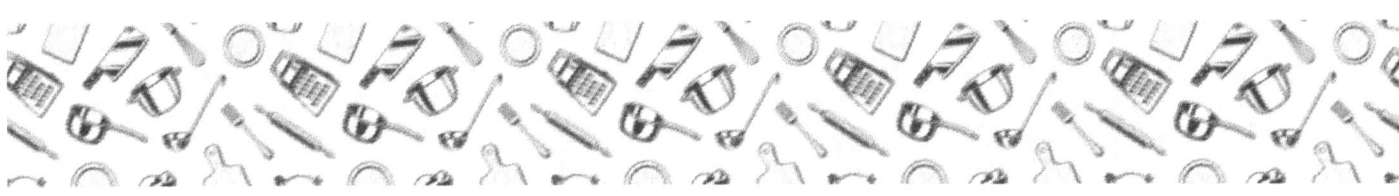

INGREDIENTS

1/2 cup chopped pecans
3 tablespoons raspberry vinegar
3 tablespoons balsamic vinegar
3 tablespoons olive oil
6 cups mixed salad greens
2 cups diced fresh strawberries
8 ounces crumbled blue cheese
1/2 cup diced red onion

Nutritional Value: 250 calories per serving

DIRECTIONS

1. Place the pecans in a skillet over medium heat. Tossing frequently, toast until lightly browned.
2. In a bowl, whisk together the raspberry vinegar, balsamic vinegar, and olive oil.
3. In a large bowl, mix the toasted pecans, greens, strawberries, blue cheese, and red

.

Salads

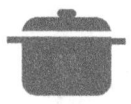 **Mixed Greens and Gorgonzola Salad**

COOKING: 10 MIN   SERVES: 2

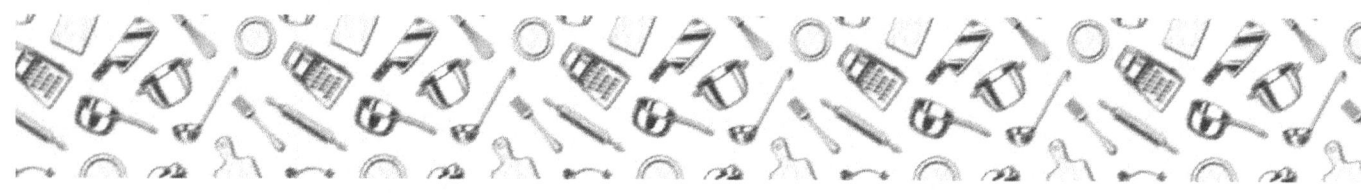

INGREDIENTS

3/4 cup walnut halves
10 ounces mixed salad greens with arugula
2 large navel oranges, peeled and sectioned
1/2 cup sliced red onion
1/4 cup olive oil
1/4 cup olive oil
2/3 cup orange juice 1/4 cup raw honey
2 tablespoons balsamic vinegar
2 teaspoons Dijon mustard
1/4 teaspoon dried oregano
1/4 teaspoon ground black pepper
1/4 cup crumbled Gorgonzola cheese

Nutritional Value: 447 calories per serving

DIRECTIONS

1. Place the walnuts in a skillet over medium heat. Cook 5 minutes, stirring constantly, until lightly browned.
2. In a large bowl, toss the toasted walnuts, salad greens, oranges, and red onion.
3. In a large jar with a lid, mix the olive oil, olive oil, orange juice, sugar, vinegar, mustard, oregano, and pepper. Seal jar and shake to mix.
4. Divide the salad greens mixture into individual servings. To serve, sprinkle with Gorgonzola cheese, and drizzle with the dressing mixture.

Salads

Eggplant Salad

COOKING: 10 MIN   SERVES: 2

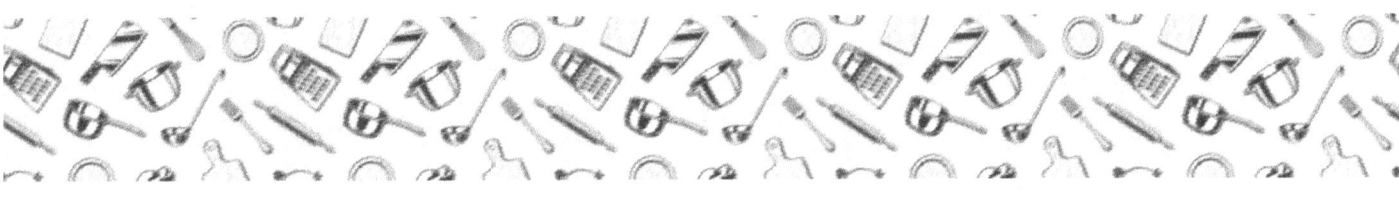

INGREDIENTS

6 eggplants
1 clove garlic, crushed
3 tablespoons olive oil
1 tablespoon balsamic vinegar
2 tablespoons raw honey
1 teaspoon dried parsley
1 teaspoon dried oregano
1/4 teaspoon dried basil salt and pepper to taste

Nutritional Value: 250 calories per serving

DIRECTIONS

1. Preheat the oven to 350 degrees F (175 degrees C). Puncture eggplants with a fork, and place on a baking sheet. Bake for 1 1/2 hours, or until soft, turning occasionally. Cool, then peel and dice.
2. In a large bowl, stir together the garlic, olive oil, vinegar, sugar, parsley, oregano, basil, salt and pepper. Add the diced eggplant and stir to coat. Refrigerate for at least 2 hours before serving to marinate.

Salads

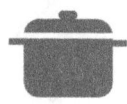 **Mandarina, Orange and Gorgonzola Salad**

COOKING: 10 MIN   SERVES: 2

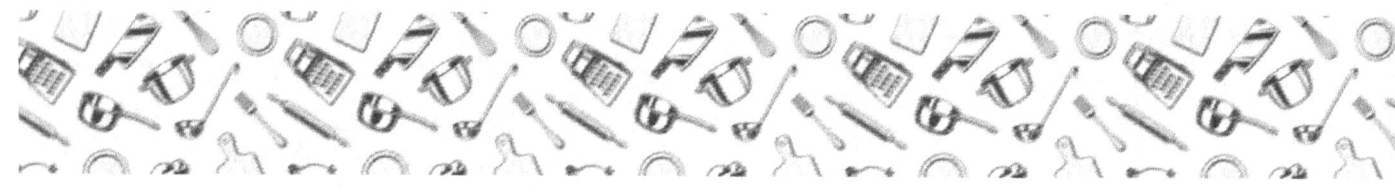

INGREDIENTS

1/2 cup blanched slivered almonds
1 (11 ounce) can mandarin oranges, juice reserved
2 tablespoons vegetable oil
2 tablespoons red wine vinegar
12 ounces mixed salad greens
1 cup Gorgonzola cheese

Nutritional Value: 354 calories per serving

DIRECTIONS

1. Heat a skillet over medium-high heat. Add almonds, and cook, stirring frequently, until lightly toasted. Remove from heat and set aside.
2. In a small bowl, whisk together 2 tablespoons reserved mandarin orange juice, oil, and vinegar.
3. In a large salad bowl, toss together the toasted almonds, mandarin oranges, mixed salad greens, and Gorgonzola cheese. Just before serving, pour dressing on salad, and toss to coat.

Salads

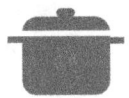

SpringSalad

COOKING: 10 MIN

SERVES: 2

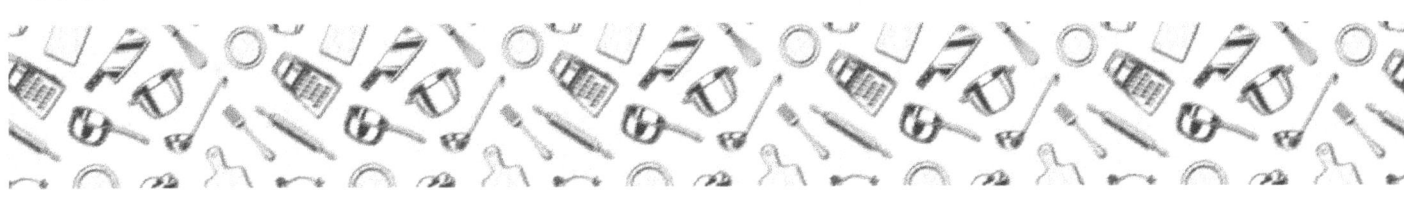

INGREDIENTS

1 bunch spinach, rinsed
10 large strawberries, sliced
1/2 cup white sugar
1 teaspoon salt
1/3 cup white wine vinegar
1 cup vegetable oil
1 tablespoon poppy seeds

Nutritional Value: 217 calories per serving

DIRECTIONS

1. In a large bowl, mix the spinach and strawberries.
2. In a blender, place the sugar, salt, vinegar, and oil, and blend until smooth. Stir in the poppy seeds. Pour over the spinach and strawberries and toss to coat.

Salads

 **Orange, Asparagus and Endive Salad**

COOKING: 10 MIN   SERVES: 2

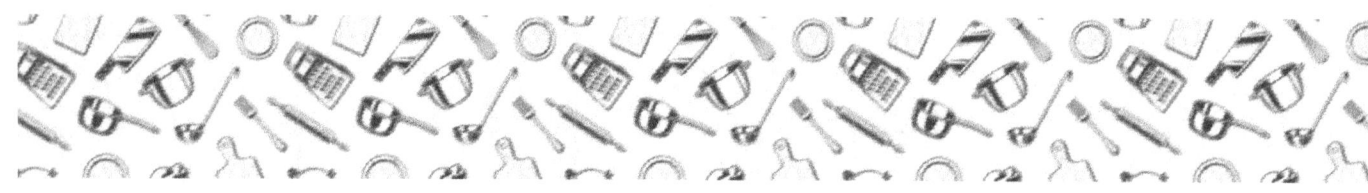

INGREDIENTS

2 1/2 cups diagonally sliced asparagus
2 cups rinsed, dried and torn endive leaves
2 large oranges, sliced into rounds
1 red onion, thinly sliced
1/3 cup raspberry vinegar
2 tablespoons canola oil
1 tablespoon orange juice
1 tablespoon raw honey salt and pepper to taste

Nutritional Value: 217 calories per serving

DIRECTIONS

1. To a large pot of boiling water, add the asparagus. Blanch for 1 minute; drain, and plunge asparagus into a bowl of cold water. Drain again and dry.
2. In a large bowl, Mix the asparagus, endive, oranges, and red onion.
3. Whisk together the raspberry vinegar, canola oil, orange juice, sugar and salt and pepper. Add dressing to the asparagus endive mixture; toss well and serve.

.

Salads

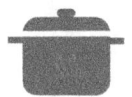

Tossed Almond Salad

COOKING: 10 MIN

SERVES: 2

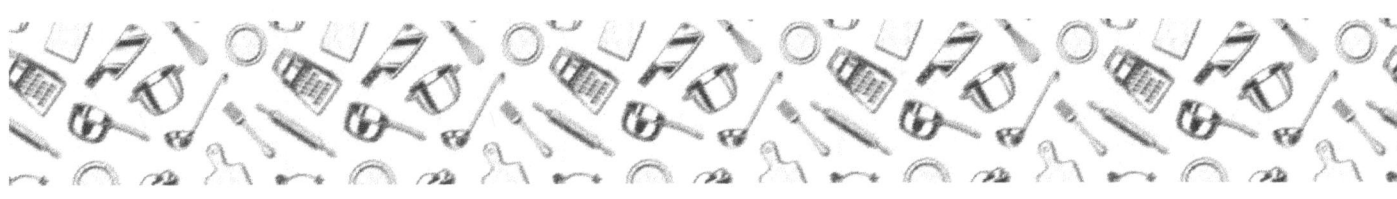

INGREDIENTS

2 tablespoons sugar
1/2 cup sliced almonds
4 cups torn iceberg lettuce
4 cups torn romaine
1 (11 ounce) can mandarin oranges, drained
1 large ripe avocado, peeled and cubed
1/2 cup diced celery
2 green onions, sliced
Dressing:
1/4 cup vegetable oil
 2 tablespoons raw honey
2 tablespoons cider vinegar
2 teaspoons minced fresh parsley
1/4 teaspoon salt
1/4 teaspoon pepper

Nutritional Value: 250 calories per serving

DIRECTIONS

1. In a small skillet over medium-low heat, cook sugar, without stirring for 12-14 minutes or until melted. Add almonds; stir quickly to coat. Remove from the heat; pour onto waxed paper to cool.
2. In a large serving bowl, combine the iceberg lettuce, romaine, oranges, avocado, celery, onions and almonds. In a jar with a tight- fitting lid, combine the dressing Ingredients; shake well. Drizzle over salad; toss gently to coat.

Salads

 **Cherry Vanilla Pear Salad**

COOKING: 10 MIN   SERVES: 2

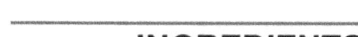

INGREDIENTS

1/4 cup white sugar
1 teaspoon ground cinnamon
1 cup walnuts
1 (15.25 ounce) can pears in light syrup, drained reserving syrup
3 tablespoons white wine vinegar
3 tablespoons fat-free vanilla yogurt
2 tablespoons honey
3/4 teaspoon kosher salt
1/4 teaspoon freshly ground black pepper
1 teaspoon vanilla extract
1 pinch ground nutmeg
1/2 (10 ounce) package mixed salad greens
1/2 (10 ounce) bag spinach leaves
1 pear - peeled, cored and sliced
1/2 cup dried cherries
1/3 cup crumbled feta cheese

Nutritional Value: 327 calories per serving

DIRECTIONS

1. Combine sugar, cinnamon and walnuts in a skillet over medium heat. Mix together until sugar and cinnamon are melted and walnuts are evenly coated. Remove from heat. Spread walnuts on a large plate to cool.
2. In the container of a blender, combine the drained pears, 1/3 cup of the reserved syrup from the can, vinegar, yogurt, honey, salt, pepper, vanilla extract, and nutmeg: blend until smooth.
3. Assemble the salad by tossing together the mixed greens, spinach, pear slices, dried cherries, feta cheese, and walnuts in a serving bowl. Serve with dressing on the side.

Salads

 **Lettuce Pear Salad**

COOKING: 10 MIN SERVES: 2

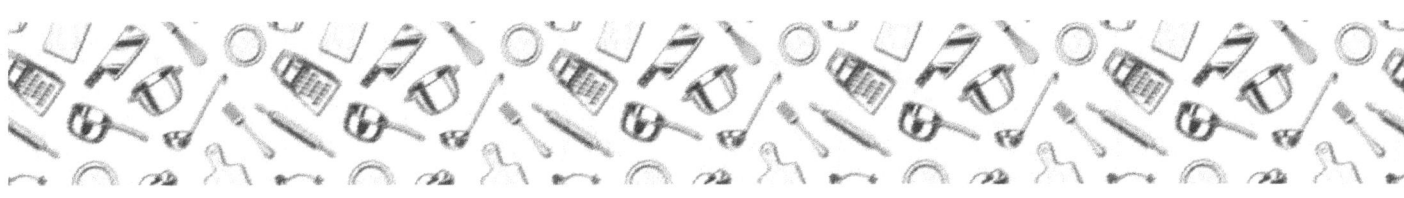

INGREDIENTS

1/2 head iceberg lettuce, torn into bite-sized pieces
1/2 cup crumbled feta cheese
1 Bosc pear, cored and cut into bite-sized pieces
1 Asian pear, cored and cut into bite-sized pieces
1/2 cup balsamic vinaigrette salad dressing

Nutritional Value: 250 calories per serving

DIRECTIONS

1. Place the lettuce into a salad bowl, sprinkle on the feta cheese in a layer, and top with a layer of Bosc and Asian pears. Serve with balsamic vinaigrette on the side.

Salads

Arugula Salad

COOKING: 10 MIN   SERVES: 2

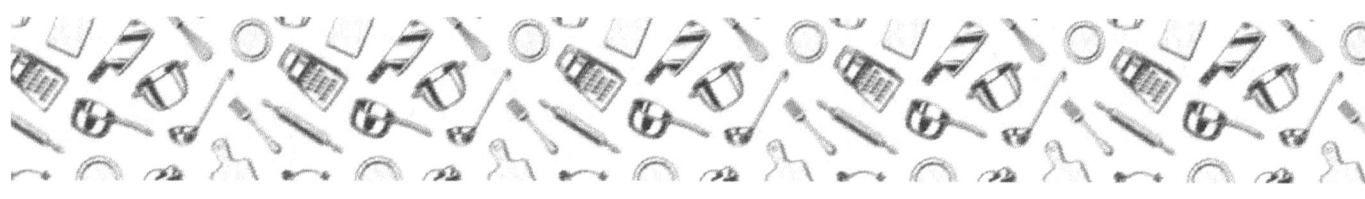

INGREDIENTS

1 tablespoon honey
1 tablespoon lemon juice
1/2 teaspoon salt
1/2 teaspoon ground black pepper
1/4 cup olive oil
1 bunch arugula
2 orange, peeled and segmented
1 bulb fennel bulb, thinly sliced
2 tablespoons sliced black olives

Nutritional Value: 350 calories per serving

DIRECTIONS

1. Whisk together the honey, lemon juice, salt, and pepper; slowly add the olive oil while continuing to whisk.
2. Place the arugula in the bottom of a salad bowl; scatter the orange segments, fennel slices, and olives over the arugula; drizzle the dressing over the salad to serve.

Salads

Creamy Orange Rice Salad

COOKING: 10 MIN

SERVES: 2

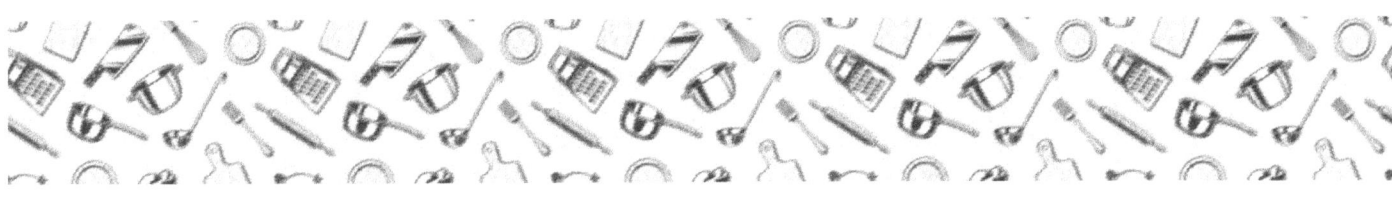

INGREDIENTS

1 teaspoon finely grated orange peel
1/2 cup orange juice
1 tablespoon finely grated fresh ginger
2 teaspoons Dijon mustard
3 tablespoons Mayonnaise
3 tablespoons extra virgin olive oil
1 1/2 cups long grain and wild rice, cooked according to package

Nutritional Value: 250 calories per serving

DIRECTIONS

1. Mix orange peel, orange juice, ginger, mustard, Hellmann's® or Best Foods® Real Mayonnaise and olive oil with wire whisk in large bowl.
2. Stir in rice, oranges, onion and parsley. Season, if desired, with salt and pepper. Sprinkle with pecans.

Salads

Beets in Orange Dressing

COOKING: 10 MIN　　　　　　　　　　　　　　SERVES: 2

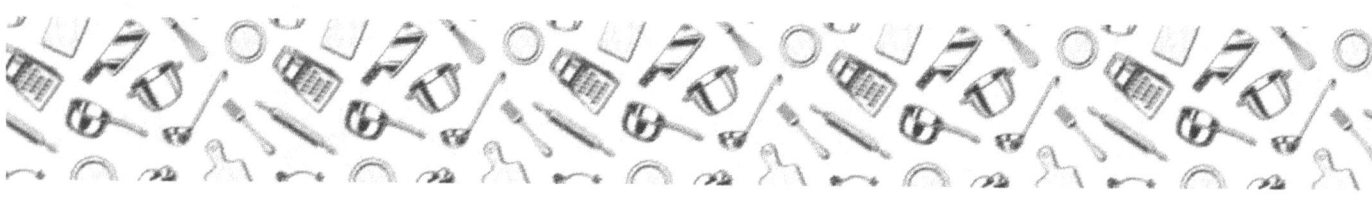

INGREDIENTS

8 medium beets
1/4 cup raw honey
2 teaspoons cornstarch Dash pepper
1 cup orange juice
1 medium navel orange, sliced and halved (optional)
1/2 teaspoon grated orange peel

Nutritional Value: 260 calories per serving

DIRECTIONS

1. Place beets in a large saucepan; cover with water. Bring to a boil. Reduce heat; cover and cook for 25-30 minutes or until tender.
2. Drain and cool slightly. Peel and slice; place in a serving bowl and keep warm.
3. In a saucepan, Mix the raw honey, cornstarch and pepper; stir in orange juice until smooth. Bring to a boil; cook and stir for 2 minutes or until thickened. Remove from the heat; stir in orange slices if desired and peel. Pour over beets.

Salads

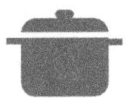

Bean Salad

COOKING: 10 MIN   SERVES: 2

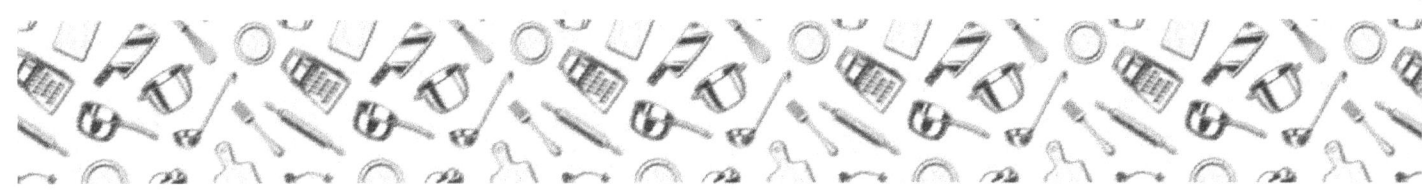

INGREDIENTS

1 (14.5 ounce) can green beans, drained
1 (14.5 ounce) can wax beans, drained
1 (15.25 ounce) can red kidney beans, drained
1 (15 ounce) can garbanzo beans, drained
1 (15 ounce) can black beans, drained
1 red onion, chopped
1 green bell pepper, chopped
3/4 cup red wine vinegar
3/4 cup white raw honey 3/4 cup olive oil
3/4 teaspoon ground dry mustard
1/2 teaspoon dried tarragon
1 1/2 teaspoons dried cilantro

Nutritional Value: 310 calories per serving

DIRECTIONS

1. In a large bowl, layer the beans, onion and green pepper. Set aside.
2. In a small saucepan, mix the vinegar, raw honey, oil, mustard, tarragon and cilantro. Cook and stir over medium heat until raw honey dissolves. Remove from heat and pour over bean mixture. Stir until all Ingredients are coated. This is best if it is left to marinate for a few hours in the refrigerator and stirred occasionally.2 teaspoons dried cilantro.

.

Salads

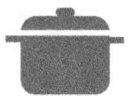

Pepper Salad

COOKING: 10 MIN   SERVES: 2

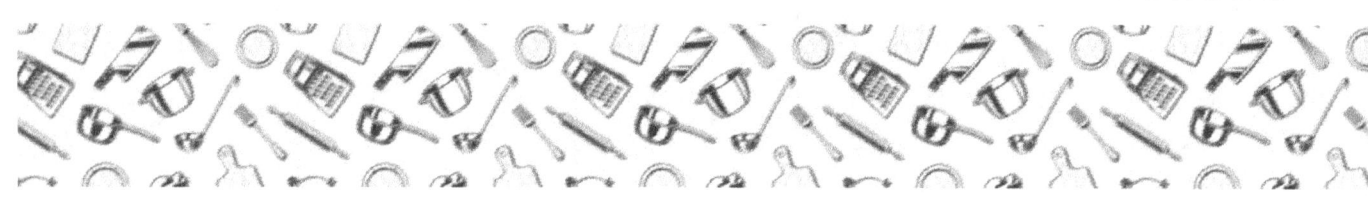

INGREDIENTS

1 1/2 (16 ounce) jars sliced pepperoncini peppers, drained
1 (32 ounce) jar sweet pepper rings, drained
1 (4 ounce) jar diced pimento peppers, drained
1-pound pepperoni sausage, cubed
1-pound provolone cheese, cubed
1/2-pound Swiss cheese, cubed
1/2-pound sharp Cheddar cheese, cubed
1 (6 ounce) can mushrooms, drained and thinly sliced
2 (6 ounce) cans black olives, drained and thinly sliced
4 cloves garlic
4 1/2 tablespoons dried oregano 1 cup canola oil
1/4 cup olive oil

Nutritional Value: 260 calories per serving

DIRECTIONS

1. In a large bowl with a lid, stir together the pepperoncini peppers, sweet pepper rings, pimentos, pepperoni, Provolone, Swiss, Cheddar, mushrooms, olives, garlic, oregano, canola oil and olive oil until evenly coated. Cover tightly with the lid and let stand in fridge for 3 days. Shake the bowl often. This can be served cold but is better when you let it come to room temperature!

Salads

Green Pea Salad

COOKING: 10 MIN   SERVES: 2

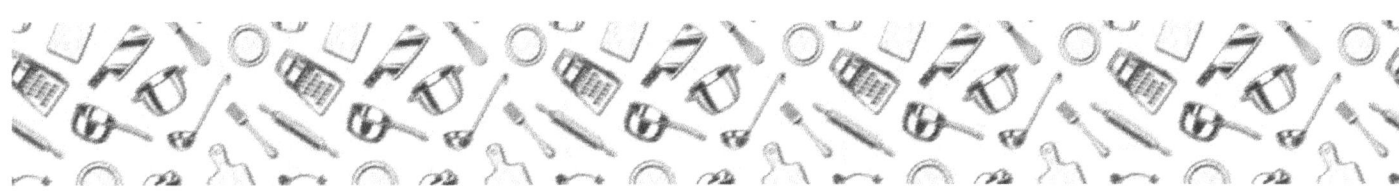

INGREDIENTS

1 (16 ounce) package frozen green peas
1 (8 ounce) can sliced water chestnuts, drained and slice into strip
6 roma (plum) tomatoes, chopped
1/2 onion, minced
2 medium sweet pickles, finely chopped
3/4 cup mayonnaise
1/8 cup lemon juice

Nutritional Value: 256 calories per serving

DIRECTIONS

1. In a colander, rinse frozen peas in cold water until thawed. Drain, and transfer to a large salad bowl.
2. Add water chestnuts, tomatoes, onion, and sweet pickles; mix well.
3. In a small bowl, mix together mayonnaise and a little pickle or lemon juice. Do not make the mixture to soupy. Pour over vegetables, and gently stir to coat.

Salads

 **Krina's Tomato Salad**

COOKING: 10 MIN　　　　　　　　　　　　　　　　　　SERVES: 2

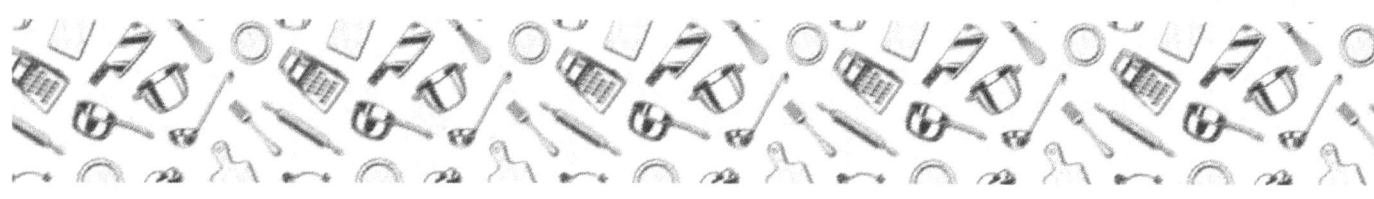

INGREDIENTS

6 plum tomatoes, chopped
1 (5 ounce) jar stuffed olives, drained and halved
3/4 cup Catalina salad dressing
1 small onion, chopped
1/4 teaspoon pepper

Nutritional Value: 310 calories per serving

DIRECTIONS

1. In a bowl, mix all Ingredients; mix well. Cover and refrigerate for at least 2 hours.

Salads

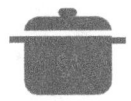

Tropical Tuna Salad

COOKING: 10 MIN   SERVES: 2

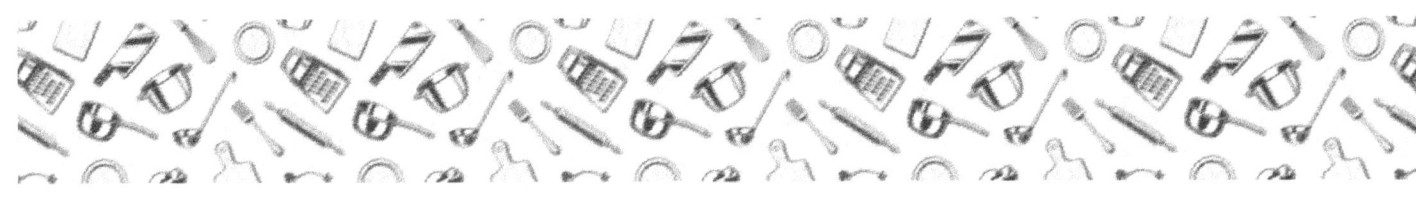

INGREDIENTS

Head romaine, torn
cups canned unsweetened pineapple chunks
1/2 cup sliced green onions
1 (12.5 ounce) can water-packed tuna, drained
1 (11 ounce) can mandarin oranges in light syrup, drained
1 (8 ounce) can sliced water chestnuts, drained
1/2 cup fat-free mayonnaise
4 teaspoons light soy sauce
1/2 teaspoon lemon juice

Nutritional Value: 369 calories per serving

DIRECTIONS

1. In a large bowl, toss romaine, pineapple, onions, tuna, oranges and water chestnuts. In a small bowl, mix mayonnaise, soy sauce and lemon juice; pour over salad and toss.

Salads

Greek Salad vol.1

COOKING: 10 MIN   SERVES: 2

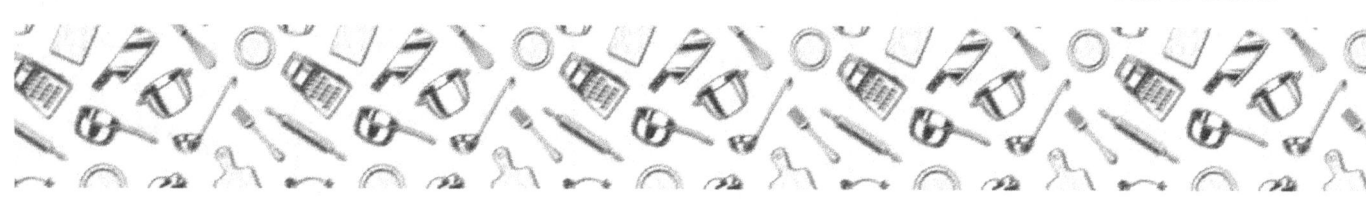

INGREDIENTS

4 large tomatoes, chopped
1 green bell pepper, chopped
1 cucumber, peeled and chopped 1 red onion, chopped
3 ounces crumbled feta cheese 1/4 cup olive oil
1/8 cup lemon juice

Nutritional Value: 136 calories per serving

DIRECTIONS

1. In a large bowl, Mix the tomatoes, green bell pepper, cucumber, red onion, olive oil, and lemon juice. Refrigerate until thoroughly chilled. Sprinkle with feta cheese before serving.

Salads

Pesto Chicken Pasta Salad

COOKING: 10 MIN   SERVES: 2

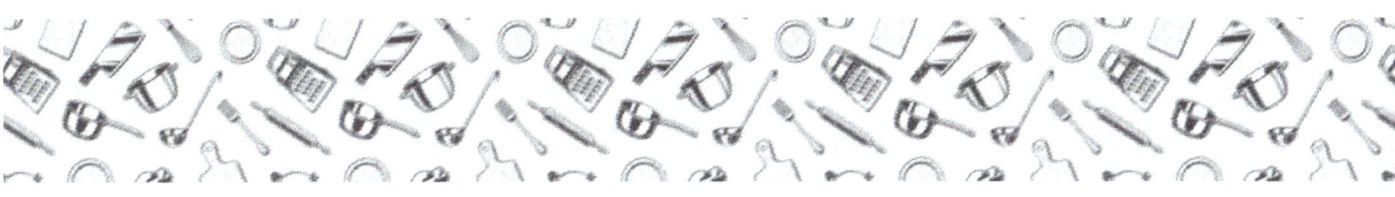

INGREDIENTS

3 heads fresh broccoli, chopped
1 red onion, chopped
3 (6 ounce) cans jumbo black olives, sliced
2 (6.5 ounce) jars marinated artichoke hearts, sliced
3 large tomatoes, chopped
3 bunches green onions, chopped
1 (8 ounce) bottle Italian-style salad dressing

Nutritional Value: 158 calories per serving

DIRECTIONS

1. In a large bowl, combine the broccoli, red onion, olives, artichoke hearts, tomatoes and green onions.
2. Add the dressing, toss, cover and refrigerate for 24 hours. The dressing will serve as a marinade and the vegetables will remain fresh, crunchy, yet easy to chew!

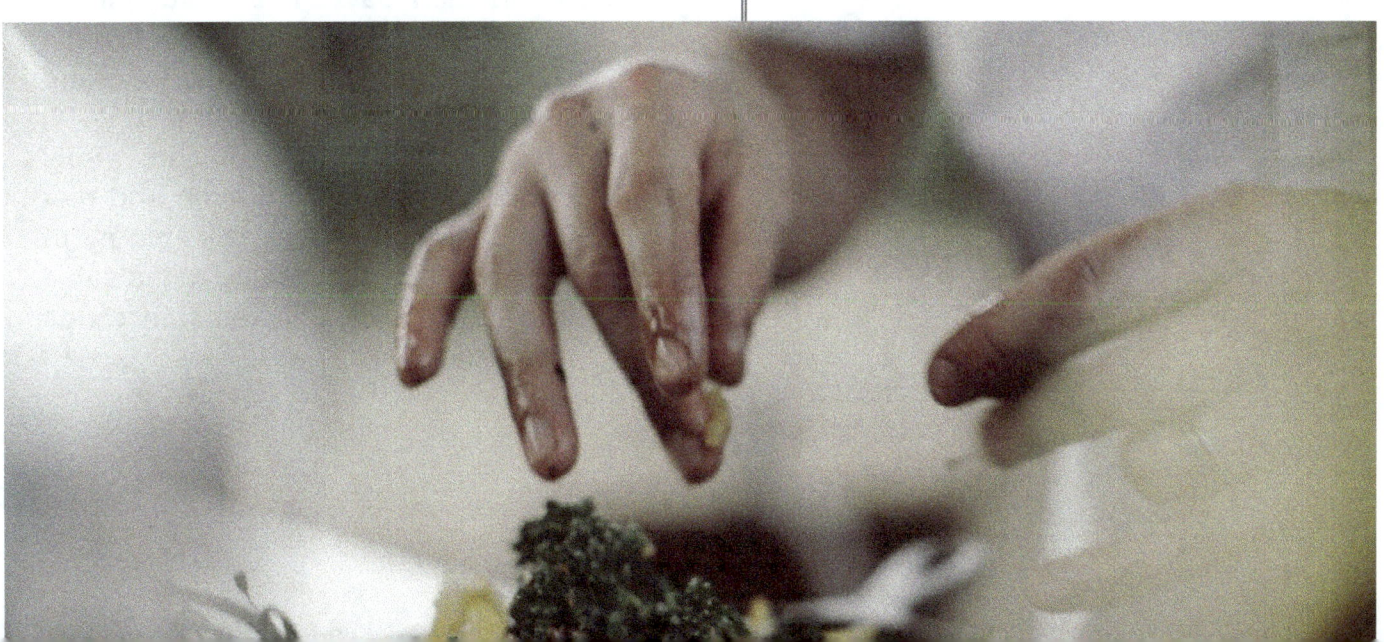

Salads

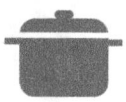 **Spinach Salad with Sesame and Ginger**

COOKING: 10 MIN   SERVES: 2

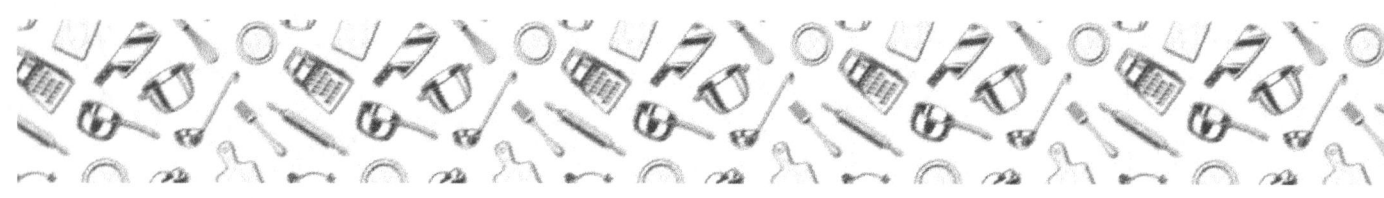

INGREDIENTS

1-pound boneless, skinless chicken breasts
1 (16 ounce) bottle Sesame Ginger Dressing
1 teaspoon black pepper
1/2 teaspoon cayenne pepper
1/2 teaspoon salt (optional)
2 tablespoons fresh herbs
6 cups baby spinach, washed, stems removed
1/2 cup raspberries, washed
1-ounce feta, crumbled
1/4 cup chopped pecans or walnuts

Nutritional Value: 168 calories per serving

DIRECTIONS

1. Preheat oven to 350 degrees F.
2. Place chicken in oven-safe baking dish. Tenderize chicken slightly with mallet or fork. Whisk together Newman's Own Lighten Up Low Fat Sesame Ginger Dressing, spices, and herbs. Pour over chicken breasts, turning breasts a couple of times. Breasts do not need to be submerged in dressing, but the dressing should fully cover the bottom of baking dish. Bake chicken 45 minutes.
3. Dry spinach leaves in a salad spinner or between two clean dish towels. Combine with raspberries, feta, and nuts in large bowl; toss to mix.
4. Once chicken breasts are fully cooked, remove from oven and rest 3 to 5 minutes. Add small amount of Newman's Own dressing to the salad and toss. Slice chicken into strips and serve over salad

Salads

Spicy Italian Salad

COOKING: 10 MIN   SERVES: 2

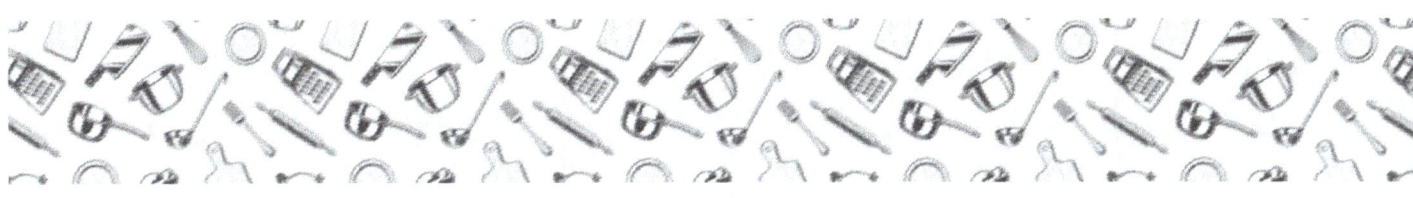

INGREDIENTS

1/2 cup canola oil
1/3 cup tarragon vinegar
1 tablespoon white sugar
1 teaspoon chopped fresh thyme
1/2 teaspoon dry mustard
2 cloves garlic, minced
1 (8 ounce) can artichoke hearts, drained and quartered
5 cups romaine lettuce - rinsed, dried, and chopped
1 red bell pepper, cut into strips
1 carrot, grated
1 red onion, thinly sliced
1/4 cup black olives
1/4 cup pitted green olives
1/2 cucumber, sliced
2 tablespoons grated Romano cheese
Pepper

Nutritional Value: 268 calories per serving

DIRECTIONS

1. In a medium container with a lid, mix canola oil, tarragon vinegar, sugar, thyme, dry mustard, and garlic. Cover, and shake until well blended. Place artichoke hearts into the mixture, cover, and marinate in the refrigerator 4 hours, or overnight.
2. In a large bowl, toss together lettuce, red bell pepper, carrot, red onion, black olives, green olives, cucumber, and Romano cheese. Season with pepper. Pour in the artichoke and marinade mixture and toss to coat.

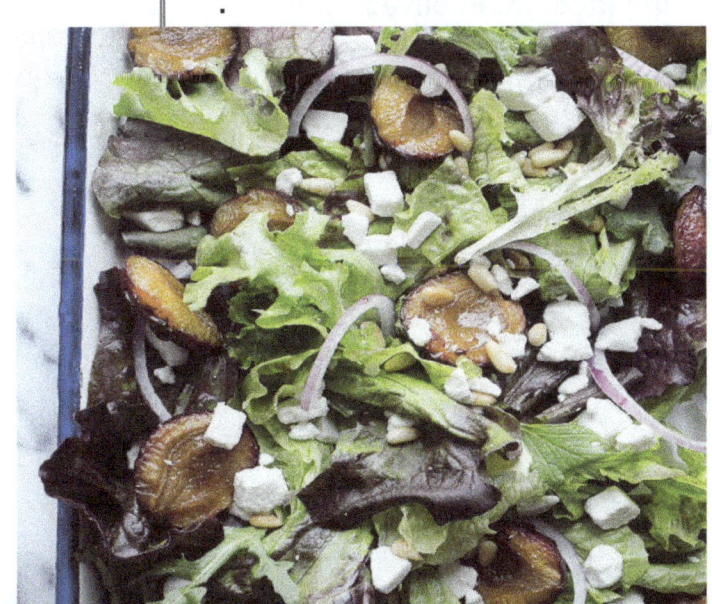

Salads

Steak and Spinach Salad

COOKING: 10 MIN

SERVES: 2

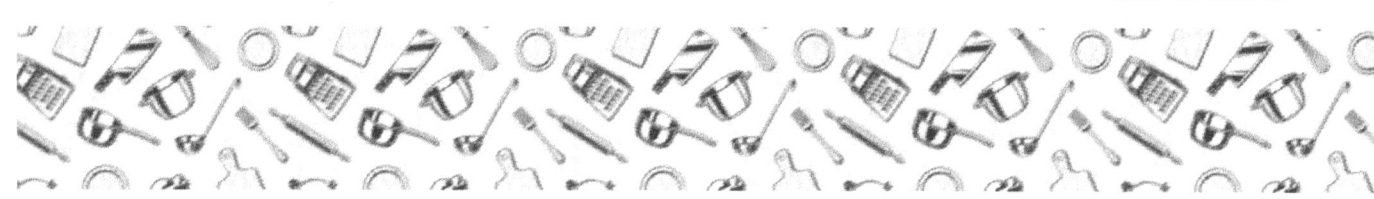

INGREDIENTS

1/2 cup canola oil
1/3 cup tarragon vinegar
1 tablespoon white sugar
1 teaspoon chopped fresh thyme
1/2 teaspoon dry mustard
2 cloves garlic, minced
1 (8 ounce) can artichoke hearts, drained and quartered
5 cups romaine lettuce - rinsed, dried, and chopped
1 red bell pepper, cut into strips
1 carrot, grated
1 red onion, thinly sliced
1/4 cup black olives
1/4 cup pitted green olives
1/2 cucumber, sliced
2 tablespoons grated Romano cheese
Pepper

Nutritional Value: 398 calories per serving

DIRECTIONS

1. Preheat an outdoor grill for medium-high heat; lightly oil the grate.
2. Season the flat iron steak on both sides with salt and pepper. Cook to desired degree of doneness on preheated grill, about 5 minutes per side for medium-rare. Let rest in a warm area while proceeding with the recipe.
3. Heat olive oil in a large skillet over medium-high heat. Stir in the onion, and cook until it begins to soften, about 4 minutes. Pour in the Italian salad dressing, and bring to a boil, then stir in the red peppers and mushrooms. Reduce heat to medium, and cook until the peppers are tender, about 5 minutes.
4. Remove the vegetables from the skillet with a slotted spoon, and set aside. Increase the heat to medium-high and add the red wine. Simmer the salad dressing and wine until it has reduced to a syrupy sauce, about 5 minutes.
5. Meanwhile, divide the spinach leaves onto serving plates. Thinly slice the flat iron steak across the grain. Spoon the warm, cooked vegetable mixture over the spinach leaves, then place the sliced steak on top. Spoon on the reduced red wine sauce, and finally, sprinkle with blue cheese.

Salads

Palms Salad

COOKING: 10 MIN

SERVES: 2

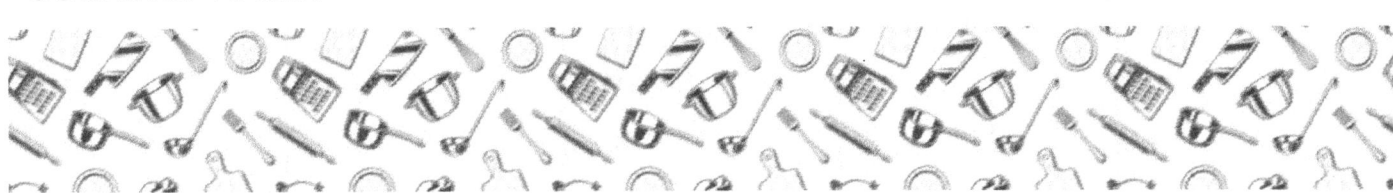

INGREDIENTS

2 (10 ounce) bags fresh spinach, rinsed and dried
1 (14.25 ounce) can hearts of palm, drained and chopped
1-pint cherry tomatoes
2 large avocados - peeled, pitted and diced
1 (10 ounce) package fresh mushrooms, sliced
1/3 cup sliced almonds
1/2 cup canola oil
1/3 cup white vinegar
1/2 cup ketchup
2 cloves garlic, chopped
1/2 cup sugar
1 teaspoon salt
1/2 teaspoon dry mustard powder
1/2 teaspoon paprika

Nutritional Value: 147 calories per serving

DIRECTIONS

1. In a large serving bowl, toss the spinach with hearts of palm, tomatoes, avocados, mushrooms, and almonds.
2. Combine oil, vinegar, ketchup, garlic and sugar in a jar. Season with salt, mustard and paprika. Cover with a tight-fitting lid. Shake vigorously until well blended.
3. Before serving, pour dressing over salad, and toss to coat evenly.

Salads

Fresh Salad

COOKING: 10 MIN SERVES: 2

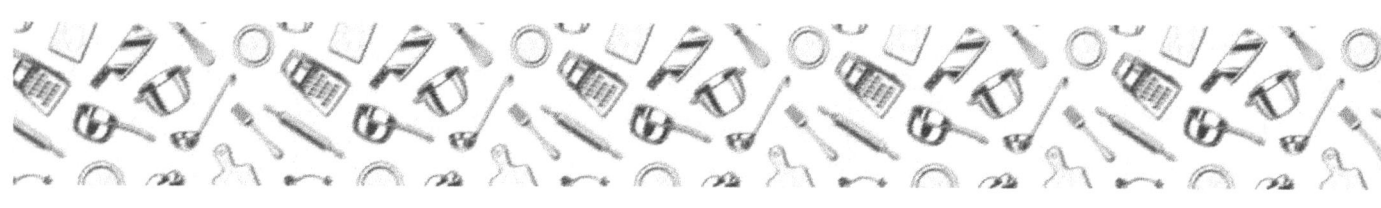

INGREDIENTS

1/2 cup white sugar
1/2 cup white vinegar
1 cup vegetable oil
2 tablespoons Worcestershire sauce
1/3 cup ketchup
1 small onion, chopped
5 slices bacon
3 eggs
1-pound fresh spinach - rinsed, dried and torn into bite size pieces
1 (4 ounce) can sliced water chestnuts, drained

Nutritional Value: 147 calories per serving

DIRECTIONS

1. In a blender or food processor, combine sugar, vinegar, oil, Worcestershire sauce, ketchup and onion, and process until smooth. Set aside.
2. Place bacon in a large, deep skillet. Cook over medium high heat until evenly brown. Drain, crumble and set aside.
3. Place eggs in a saucepan and cover with cold water. Bring water to a boil and immediately remove from heat. Cover and let eggs stand in hot water for 10 to 12 minutes. Remove from hot water, cool, peel and chop.
4. In a large bowl, toss together the spinach, water chestnuts, bacon and eggs. Serve with the dressing.

Salads

Eggplant Yogurt Salad

COOKING: 10 MIN

SERVES: 2

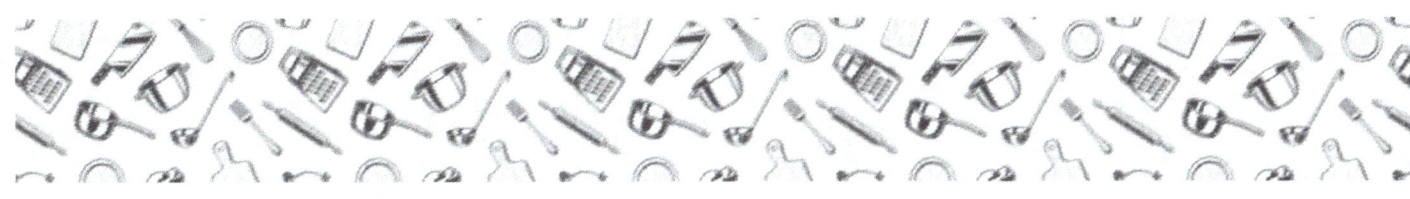

INGREDIENTS

1 medium eggplant, cubed
1/2 cup water
1 1/2 cups plain yogurt
1 bunch green onions, chopped
1/2 bunch cilantro, finely chopped
1 teaspoon ground black pepper
salt to taste
1/4 teaspoon paprika
1 tablespoon olive oil

Nutritional Value: 258 calories per serving

DIRECTIONS

1. In a pot over medium heat, add the eggplant and water; cook until tender and the water evaporates. Mash the eggplant so no large chunks remain. Allow to cool completely.
2. In a large bowl, add the yogurt, mashed eggplant, green onions, cilantro, pepper and salt; mix well.
3. To smoke the salad, heat one-piece charcoal over open flame until gray and reddish in color. Place a small square of aluminum foil in the eggplant salad (make room in the center for the foil). Place the hot charcoal on the piece of foil in the bowl. Add the olive oil on top of the charcoal and cover salad bowl immediately. Allow to smoke for 10 minutes; remove charcoal.
4. Chill the salad in the refrigerator and garnish with fresh chopped cilantro and sprinkle of paprika.

Salads

Pear Salad

COOKING: 10 MIN

SERVES: 2

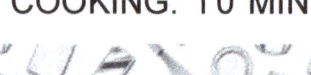

INGREDIENTS

2 firm ripe pears, halved and cored
4 teaspoons olive oil, divided
2 tablespoons cider vinegar
1 teaspoon water
1 teaspoon honey
1/4 teaspoon salt
1/8 teaspoon white pepper
1 (10 ounce) package mixed baby salad greens
1 cup watercress sprigs
1/4 cup chopped toasted hazelnuts
1/4 cup dried cranberries

Nutritional Value: 241 calories per serving

DIRECTIONS

1. In a bowl, toss pears with 1 teaspoon oil. Place in a 15-in. x 10-in. x 1-in. baking pan coated with nonstick cooking spray. Bake at 400 degrees F for 10 minutes. Turn pears over; bake 5-7 minutes longer or until golden and tender.
2. When cool enough to handle, peel pears. Thinly slice two pear halves lengthwise and set aside. Place remaining pear halves in a food processor or blender. Add the vinegar, water, honey, salt and white pepper, cover and process until smooth. While processing, slowly add remaining oil.
3. In a large bowl, toss the salad greens, watercress, nuts and cranberries. Arrange pear slices on top, drizzle with dressing.

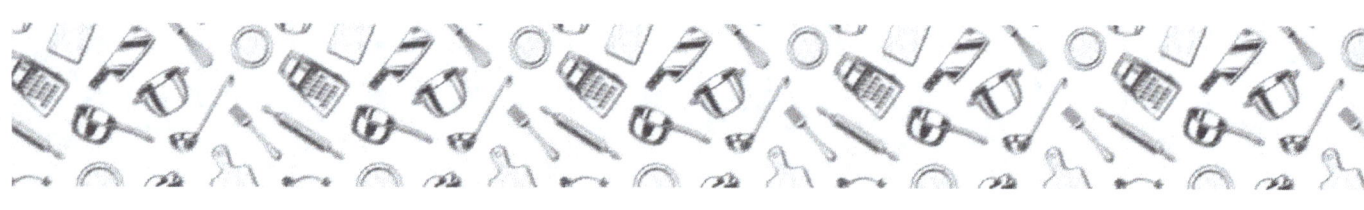

Salads

Chicken Salad with Pecans

COOKING: 10 MIN SERVES: 2

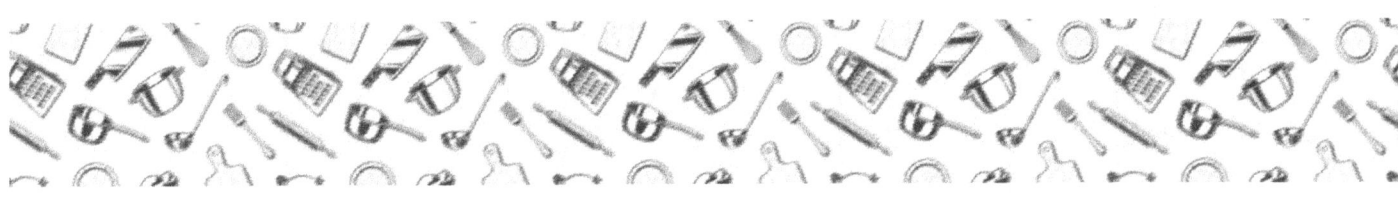

INGREDIENTS

1 cup creamy garlic salad dressing
1 cup finely chopped pecans
4 skinless, boneless chicken breast halves
1 head romaine lettuce leaves, torn into
1/2-inch-wide strips
1 (15 ounce) can mandarin oranges, drained
1 cup dried cranberries
4 ounces blue cheese, crumbled
1/2 cup Ranch dressing

Nutritional Value: 269 calories per serving

DIRECTIONS

1. Preheat oven to 400 degrees F (200 degrees C).
2. Place the creamy garlic dressing and pecans in separate bowls. Dip each chicken breast in the dressing then in the pecans to coat.
3. Arrange chicken on a baking sheet.
4. Bake chicken 25 minutes in the preheated oven, until juices run clear. Cool slightly and cut into strips.
4. On serving plates, arrange equal amounts of the lettuce, mandarin oranges, cranberries, and blue cheese. Top with equal amounts chicken and serve with Ranch dressing
.

Salads

 Rice, Pecans and Chicken Salad

COOKING: 10 MIN SERVES: 2

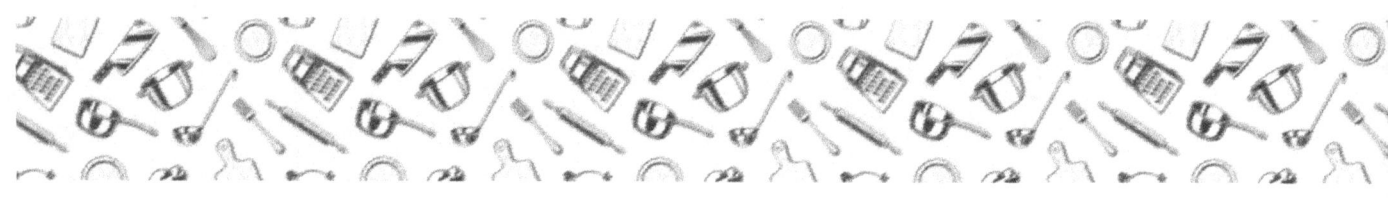

INGREDIENTS

4 (4 ounce) skinless, boneless chicken breasts
3 1/2 cups cooked wild rice
1 cup sliced green grapes
1 cup sliced green onions (optional)
1/4 cup chopped pecans, toasted (optional)
1 tablespoon grated pecans, toasted (optional)
1 tablespoon grated orange rind
1 cup Orange Marmalade
1/3 cup raspberry vinegar
1/4 teaspoon salt
1/8 teaspoon pepper
Cooking Spray

Nutritional Value: 352 calories per serving

DIRECTIONS

1. Spray a large skillet with Crisco cooking spray: heat over medium-high heat until hot. Add chicken; cook 2 minutes on each side or until lightly browned.
2. Place chicken in an 11x17-inch baking dish coated with cooking spray. Bake at 450 for 20 minutes or until cooked through. Remove chicken: cook and cut into 1/4-inch strips.
3. In a large bowl, combine chicken, rice, green onions, and grapes and pecans, if desired. Toss well and set aside. In a small bowl, combine orange rind and next 4 Ingredients; stir well. Pour over chicken mixture; toss well.
4. Serve salad at room temperature, on lettuce-lined plates, if desired.

Salads

Honey Tenderloin Salad

COOKING: 10 MIN SERVES: 2

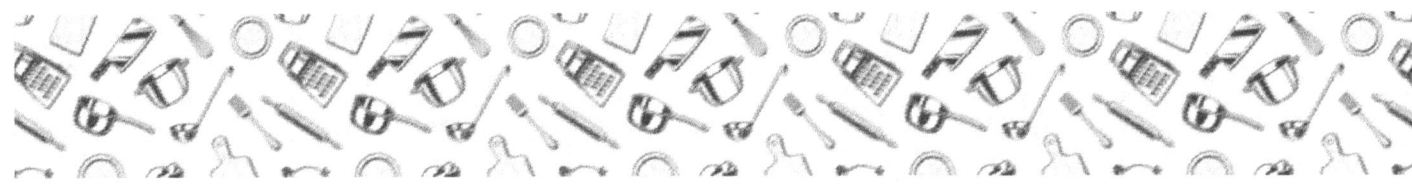

INGREDIENTS

4 (4 ounce) beef tenderloin steaks, cut 3/4 inch thick
1/2 teaspoon coarse grind black pepper
1 (5 ounce) package mixed baby salad greens
1 medium red or green pear, cored, cut into wedges
1/4 cup dried cranberries Salt
1/4 cup coarsely chopped pecans, toasted
1/4 cup crumbled goat cheese (optional)
Honey Mustard Dressing:
1/2 cup prepared honey mustard
2 tablespoons water
1 1/2 teaspoons olive oil
1 teaspoon white wine vinegar
1/4 teaspoon coarse grind black pepper
1/8 teaspoon salt

Nutritional Value: 250 calories per serving

DIRECTIONS

1. Season beef steaks with 1/2 teaspoon pepper. Heat large nonstick skillet over medium heat until hot. Place steaks in skillet; cook 7 to 9 minutes for medium rare (145 degrees F) to medium (160 degrees F) doneness, turning occasionally.
2. Meanwhile whisk Honey Mustard Dressing Ingredients in small bowl until well blended. Set aside. Divide greens evenly among 4 plates. Top evenly with pear wedges and dried cranberries.
3. Carve steaks into thin slices, season with salt as desired. Divide steak slices evenly over salads. Top each salad evenly with dressing, pecans and goat cheese, if desired.

Salads

Apple Salad

COOKING: 10 MIN

SERVES: 2

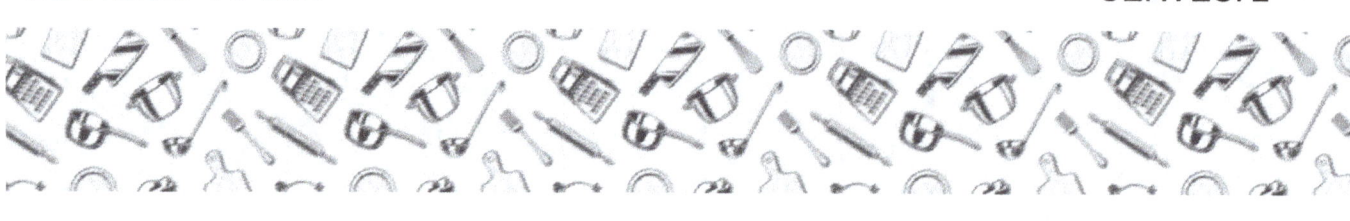

INGREDIENTS

1 cup baby spinach leaves
1 tablespoon dried cranberries
1 tablespoon chopped salted pecans
1/2 apple, cored and diced
1 tablespoon diced red onion
2 tablespoons grated carrot
1/4 avocado, peeled and diced
1 tablespoon balsamic vinaigrette salad dressing, or to taste

Nutritional Value: 270 calories per serving

DIRECTIONS

1. Place spinach, cranberries, pecans, apple, onion, carrot, and avocado into a bowl. Drizzle with balsamic vinaigrette and toss to coat.

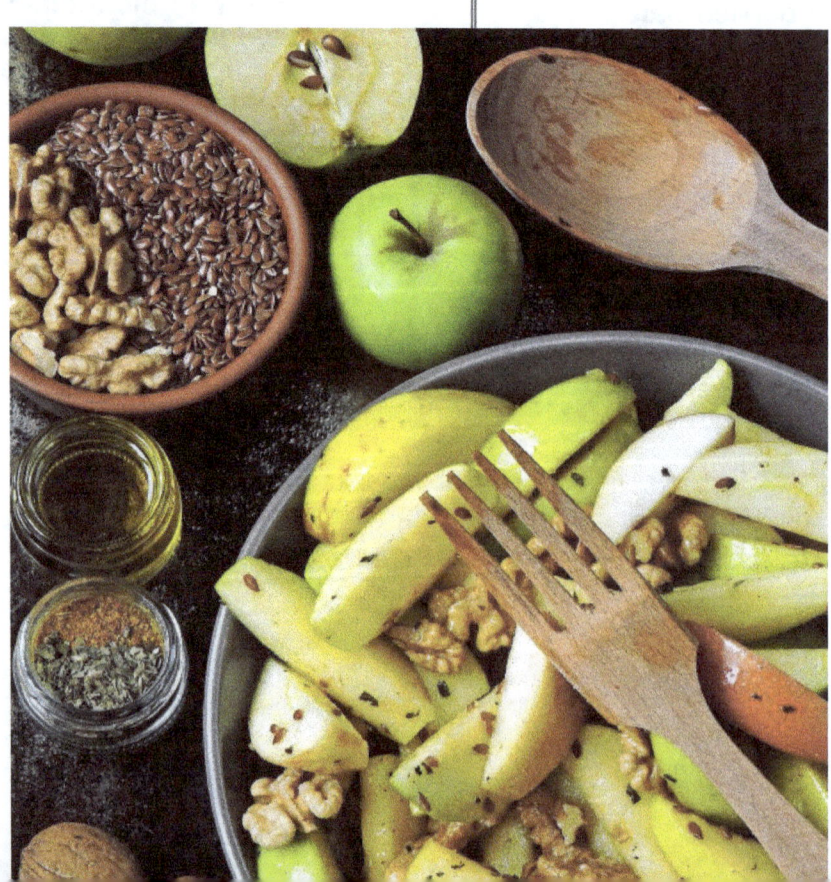

Salads

Pears and Ricotta Salad

COOKING: 10 MIN

SERVES: 2

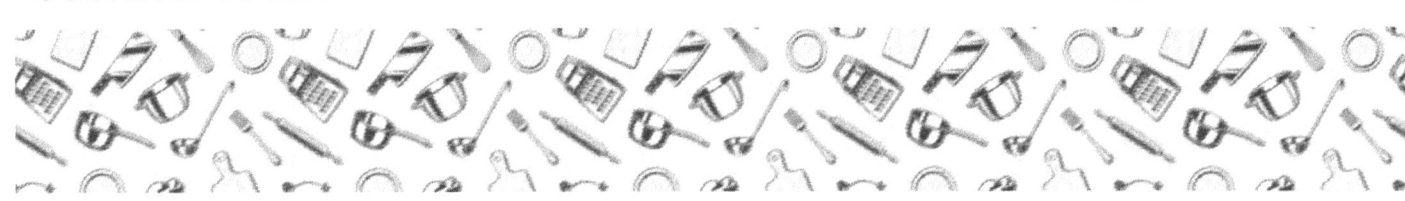

INGREDIENTS

Sherry Vinaigrette:
1/4 cup sherry vinegar
1/2 teaspoon whole grain Dijon mustard
Sea salt to taste
Fresh cracked pepper to taste
1/2 packet stevia
1/4 cup extra virgin olive oil
Roasted Pears and Ricotta Salata:
4 medium Bosc pears or any winter or summer pears, peeled and cut into 8 wedges
1 (3 ounce) chunk ricotta
1 1/2 tablespoons extra virgin olive oil
Salt
Pepper
12-inch preheated sheet pan or large sauté pan
Small head radicchio

Nutritional Value: 256 calories per serving

DIRECTIONS

1. *Sherry Vinaigrette:* Combine vinegar, mustard, sea salt, pepper with Stevia Extract In The Raw. Whisk vigorously to dissolve. Add extra virgin olive oil and whisk in until incorporated. Set aside.
2. *Roasted Pears and Ricotta:* Preheat oven to 450 degrees F and place rack in middle position in oven.
3. Toss the cut pears in the olive oil, sea salt and pepper.
4. Carefully remove preheated sheet pan or saute pan from oven and spread pears out. Quickly put pears back into oven to roast approximately 5 minutes. They should be soft but maintain firmness. Remove from oven and set aside on rack to cool.
5. Shave ricotta.
5. Place pears and cheese on radicchio and serve
.

Salads

Tarragon Salad

COOKING: 10 MIN

SERVES: 2

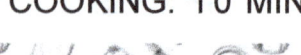

INGREDIENTS

1 bunch spinach, rinsed and torn into bite-size pieces
2 eggs
5 slices bacon
1/2 cup vegetable oil
2 tablespoons red wine vinegar
1 teaspoon white sugar
1/2 teaspoon salt
1/2 teaspoon dried tarragon
1/4 teaspoon ground black pepper

Nutritional Value: 239 calories per serving

DIRECTIONS

1. Place eggs in a saucepan and cover with cold water. Bring water to a boil. Cover, remove from heat, and let eggs stand in hot water for 10 to 12 minutes. Remove from hot water, and cool, peel and chop.
2. Place bacon in a large, deep skillet. Cook over medium high heat until evenly brown. Drain, crumble and set aside.
3. Combine the spinach, egg and bacon.
4. Whisk together the oil, vinegar, sugar, salt, tarragon and pepper. Pour enough dressing over salad to coat; toss and serve.

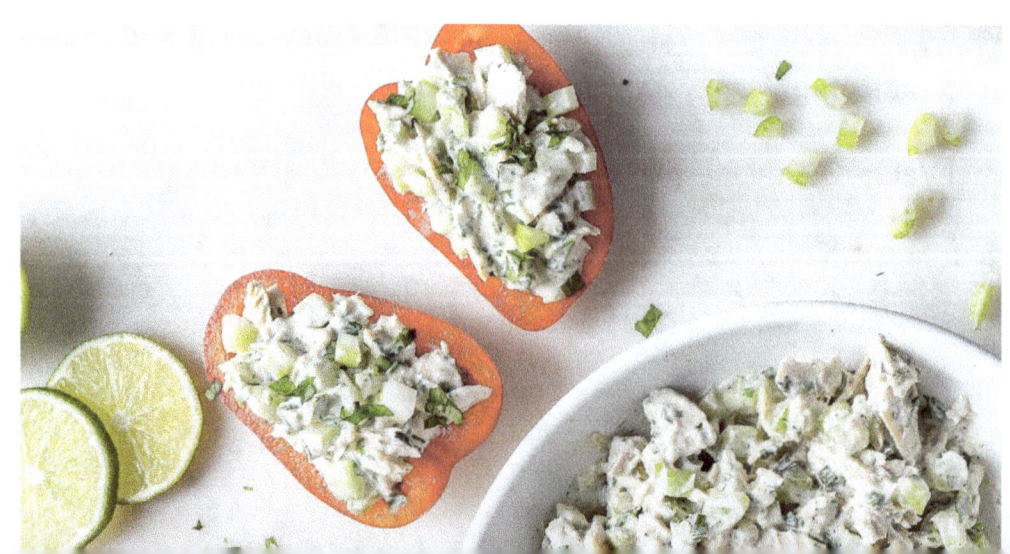

Salads

Blue Cheese and Pear Salad

COOKING: 10 MIN   SERVES: 2

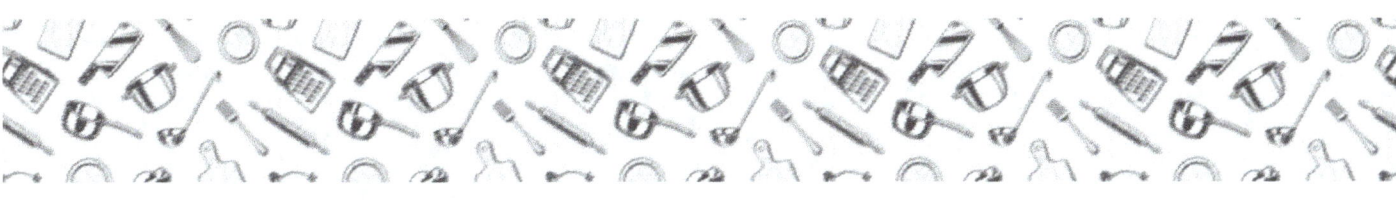

INGREDIENTS

1 (10 ounce) bag mixed field greens
1/2 cup sliced red onion (optional)
1 Bosc pear, cored and sliced
1/2 cup chopped candied pecans
1/2 cup crumbled blue cheese
1/4 cup maple syrup
1/3 cup apple cider vinegar
1/2 cup mayonnaise
2 tablespoons packed brown sugar
3/4 teaspoon salt
1/4 teaspoon freshly ground black pepper
1/4 cup walnut oil

Nutritional Value: 320 calories per serving

DIRECTIONS

1. Place the salad greens in a large bowl. Add the red onion, pear, pecans, and blue cheese, and toss to mix evenly.
2. To make the dressing, place the maple syrup, vinegar, mayonnaise, brown sugar, salt, and pepper in a blender, and blend thoroughly.
3. With the motor running, slowly pour in the walnut oil. Blend until mixture becomes creamy, about 1 minute. Pour over salad mixture and toss to coat greens evenly. Serve immediately.

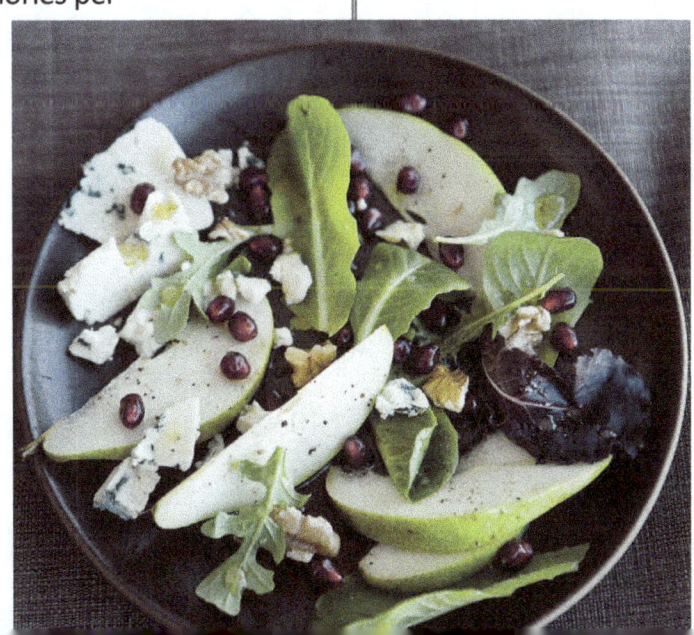

Salads

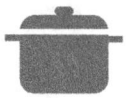

Tossed Salad

COOKING: 10 MIN

SERVES: 2

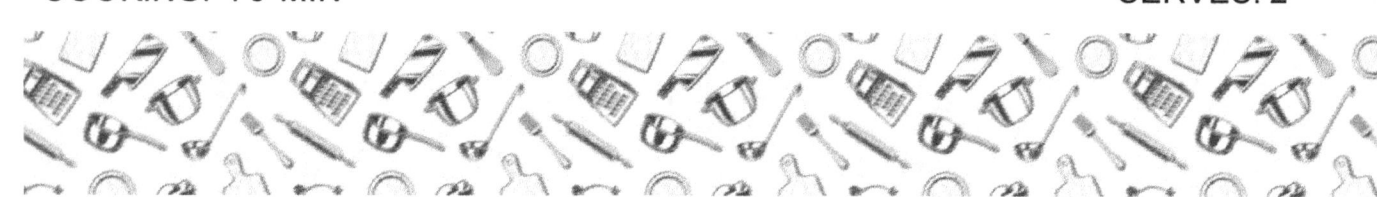

INGREDIENTS

2 tablespoons sugar
1/2 cup sliced almonds
4 cups torn iceberg lettuce
4 cups torn romaine
1 (11 ounce) can mandarin oranges, drained
1 large ripe avocado, peeled and cubed
1/2 cup diced celery
2 green onions, sliced
Dressing:
1/4 cup olive oil
2 tablespoons sugar
2 tablespoons cider vinegar
2 teaspoons minced fresh parsley
1/4 teaspoon salt
1/4 teaspoon pepper

Nutritional Value: 257 calories per serving

DIRECTIONS

1. In a small skillet over medium-low heat, cook sugar, without stirring for 12-14 minutes or until melted. Add almonds; stir quickly to coat. Remove from the heat; pour onto waxed paper to cool.
2. In a large serving bowl, Mix the iceberg lettuce, romaine, oranges, avocado, celery, onions and almonds. In a jar with a tight-fitting lid, Mix the dressing Ingredients; shake well. Drizzle over salad; toss gently to coat.

Salads

Salad with Nuts

COOKING: 10 MIN

SERVES: 2

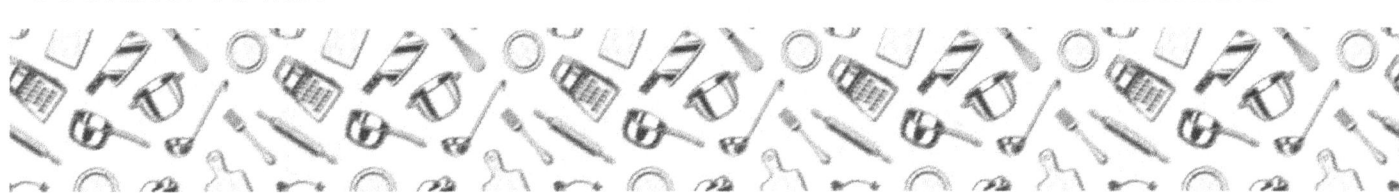

INGREDIENTS

1/4 cup apple cider vinegar
1/4 cup sugar
1/4 cup vegetable oil
1/4 teaspoon paprika
1 dash Worcestershire sauce
1 tablespoon butter
½ cup slivered almonds
1-quart strawberries
2 romaine hearts, chopped into bite size pieces

Nutritional Value: 199 calories per serving

DIRECTIONS

1. In a bowl, mix the vinegar, sugar, oil, paprika, and Worcestershire sauce. Cover, and refrigerate at least 6 hours.
2. Melt butter in a skillet over medium heat. Stir in the almonds and cook until golden brown. Remove from heat, and cool.
3. In a bowl, toss the strawberries, romaine, and almonds. Mix with the dressing just before serving.

Salads

 **Feta Strawberry Salad**

COOKING: 10 MIN SERVES: 2

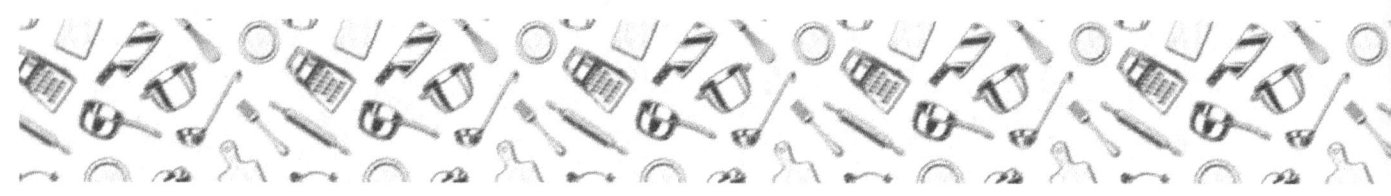

INGREDIENTS

1 cup slivered almonds
2 cloves garlic, minced 1 teaspoon honey
1 teaspoon Dijon mustard
1/4 cup raspberry vinegar
2 tablespoons balsamic vinegar
2 tablespoons brown sugar
1 cup vegetable oil
1 head romaine lettuce, torn
1-pint fresh strawberries, sliced
1 cup crumbled feta cheese

Nutritional Value: 235 calories per serving

DIRECTIONS

1. In a skillet over medium-high heat, cook the almonds, stirring frequently, until lightly toasted. Remove from heat and set aside.
2. In a bowl, prepare the dressing by whisking together the garlic, honey, Dijon mustard, raspberry vinegar, balsamic vinegar, brown sugar, and vegetable oil.
3. In a large bowl, toss together the toasted almonds, romaine lettuce, strawberries, and feta cheese. Cover with the dressing mixture and toss to serve.

Salads

 Red Potato Salad

COOKING: 10 MIN   SERVES: 2

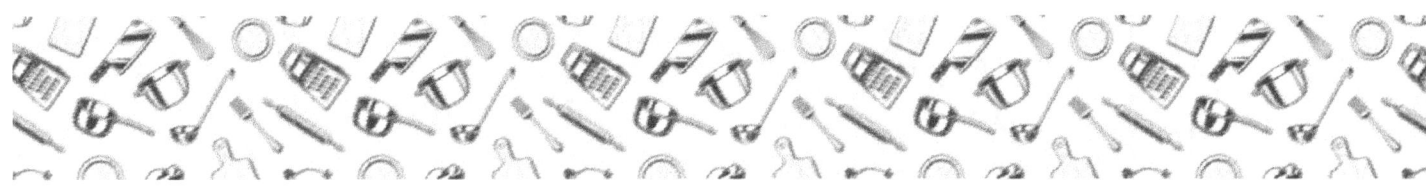

INGREDIENTS

18 small red potatoes
3 pounds fresh asparagus, trimmed
2 (14 ounce) cans artichoke hearts, drained and quartered
3 tablespoons Dijon mustard
1/4 cup fresh lemon juice
3/4 cup olive oil
salt and ground black pepper to taste
1/4 teaspoon cayenne pepper, or to taste
5 tablespoons minced fresh chives

Nutritional Value: 250 calories per serving

DIRECTIONS

1. Place the potatoes into a large pot and cover with salted water. Bring to a boil over high heat, then reduce heat to medium-low, cover, and simmer until tender, about 20 minutes. Drain and allow to steam dry for a minute or two. Allow to cool completely before cutting into bite-size cubes. Transfer to a large bowl
2. Bring a large pot of salted water to a boil over high heat. Add the asparagus spears, and cook until tender, about 3 minutes depending on size. Drain and immediately plunge into cold water to stop cooking. Cut the asparagus spears into 1-inch pieces. Place in the bowl with the potatoes. Stir in the artichokes, breaking them apart slightly as you put them in the bowl.
3. Combine the mustard and lemon juice in a bowl; whisk the oil gradually into the mustard and lemon juice until smooth. Season with salt, pepper, and cayenne pepper to taste. Drizzle over the vegetables; toss to coat. Sprinkle with chives to serve.

Salads

Chicken Salad with Peaches

COOKING: 10 MIN   SERVES: 2

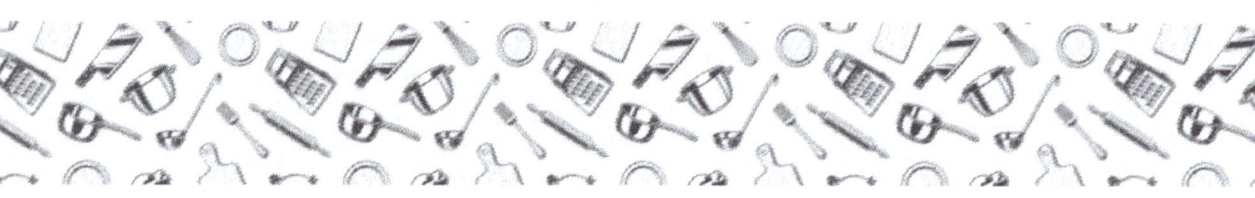

INGREDIENTS

3 medium fresh peaches, peeled and cubed
2 cups cubed cooked chicken breast
1 medium cucumber, seeded and chopped
3 tablespoons finely chopped red onion
Vinaigrette:
1/4 cup white wine vinegar
1 tablespoon lemon juice
1/3 cup sugar
1/4 cup minced fresh mint
1/4 teaspoon salt
1/8 teaspoon pepper
4 lettuce leaves

Nutritional Value: 258 calories per serving

DIRECTIONS

1. In a large bowl, combine the peaches, chicken, cucumber and onion; set aside. In a blender, combine the vinegar, lemon juice, sugar, mint, salt and pepper, cover and process until smooth.
2. Drizzle over chicken mixture; toss to coat. Cover and refrigerate until chilled. Use a slotted spoon to serve on lettuce-lined plates.

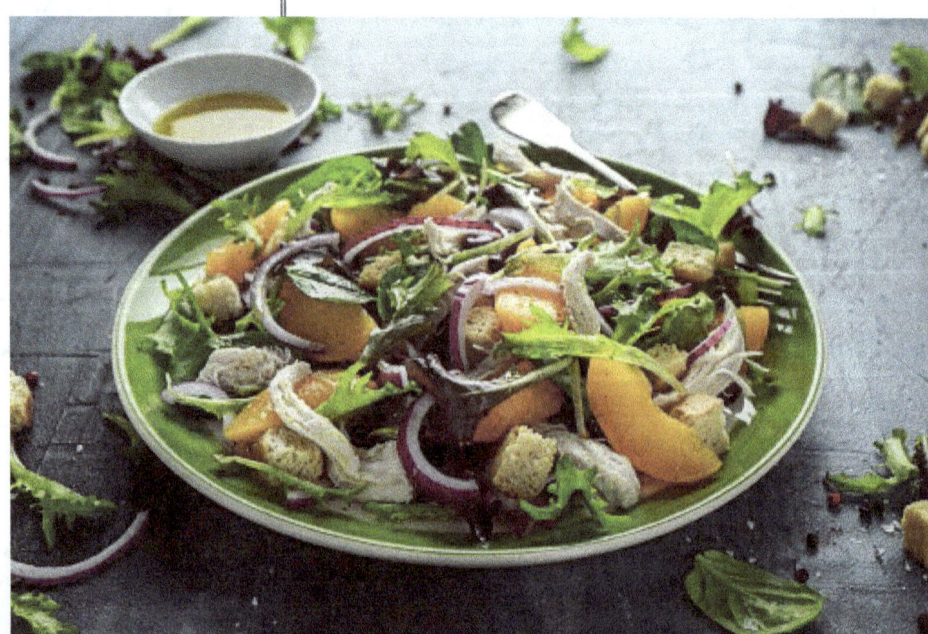

Salads

Orange and Mushroom Salad

COOKING: 10 MIN   SERVES: 2

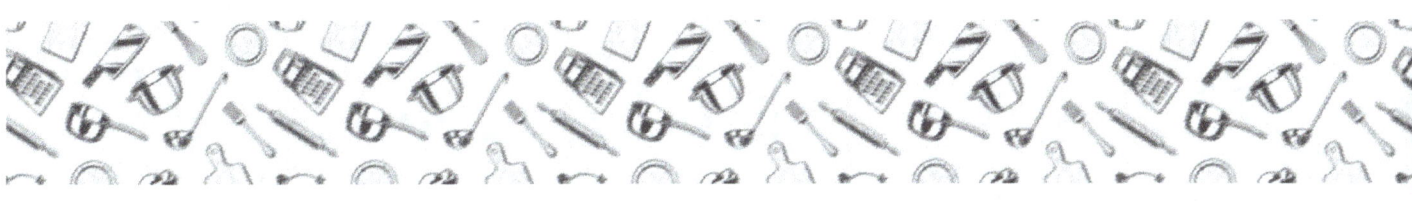

INGREDIENTS

8 ounces bacon, slice into 1-inch pieces
3/4 cup orange juice
1/4 cup shallots, minced
1/4 cup olive oil
1/4 cup balsamic vinegar
4 large oranges, peeled and segmented
10 ounces spinach, rinsed and chopped
1 medium head radicchio
6 ounces fresh shiitake mushrooms, stemmed and sliced
6 ounces fresh oyster mushrooms, stemmed and sliced
1/2 cup chopped toasted hazelnuts
1 (3 ounce) package enoki mushrooms

Nutritional Value:

250 calories per serving

DIRECTIONS

1. Place bacon in a large, deep skillet. Cook over medium high heat until evenly brown. Remove, crumble and set aside. Reserve bacon fat.
2. Whisk together 1/4 cup bacon fat, orange juice, shallots, olive oil and vinegar.
3. In a large bowl, Mix the spinach and radicchio.
4. Heat 2 tablespoons reserved bacon drippings in skillet over medium-high heat. Add shitake mushrooms and cook for 1 minute. Add oyster mushrooms and cook for 2 minutes. Season with salt and pepper; add to greens and toss.
5. Pour dressing into same skillet and boil 2 minutes. Pour dressing over greens. Add bacon, orange segments and chopped hazelnuts. Toss to Mix. Season to taste with salt and pepper. Garnish salad with enoki mushrooms and serve.

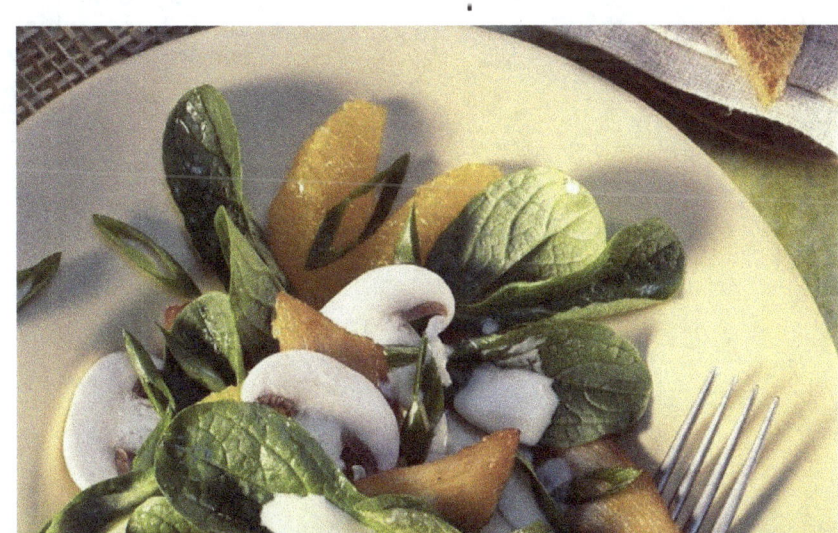

Salads

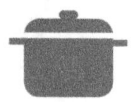

Couscous Bacon Salad

COOKING: 10 MIN

SERVES: 2

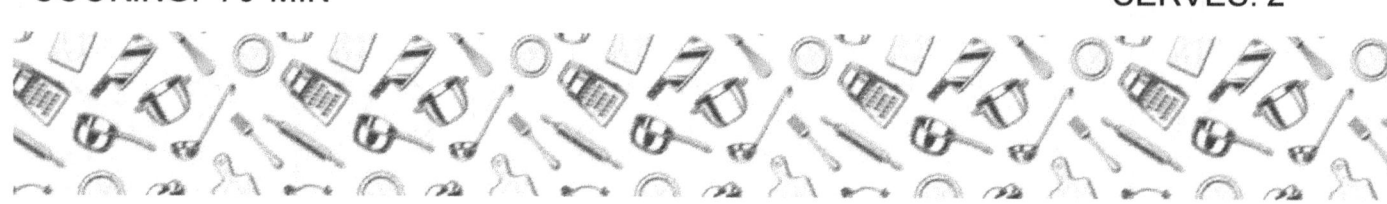

INGREDIENTS

1 (10 ounce) bag fresh spinach, rinsed and dried
4 cooked skinless, boneless chicken breast halves, sliced
1 zucchini, halved lengthwise and sliced
1 red bell pepper, chopped
1/2 cup black olives
3 ounces fontina cheese, shredded
1/2 cup fat-free roasted garlic salad dressing

Nutritional Value: 156 calories per serving

DIRECTIONS

1. Place the bacon in a large, deep skillet, and cook over medium-high heat, turning occasionally, until evenly browned, about 10 minutes. Drain the bacon slices on a paper towel-lined plate. When cool, crumble the bacon slices, and set aside.
2. Drain all but 1 tablespoon of bacon drippings from the skillet and cook and stir the onion in the skillet until the edges of the onion begin to turn brown. Set the onion aside.
3. Bring the water to a boil in a saucepan, and sprinkle in the couscous. Remove the pan from the heat, let stand for 5 minutes to absorb the water, then fluff the couscous with a fork. Allow couscous to cool.
4. Place the onion, cooled couscous, carrot, cucumber, red bell pepper, and garbanzos into a salad bowl, and stir lightly to Mix.
5. In a bowl, whisk together the olive oil, white balsamic vinegar, soy sauce, raw honey, curry powder, and salt and pepper until the raw honey has dissolved. Pour the dressing over the salad, mix again lightly, and sprinkle with bacon bits.

Salads

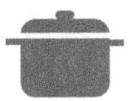

Grape Salad

COOKING: 10 MIN SERVES: 2

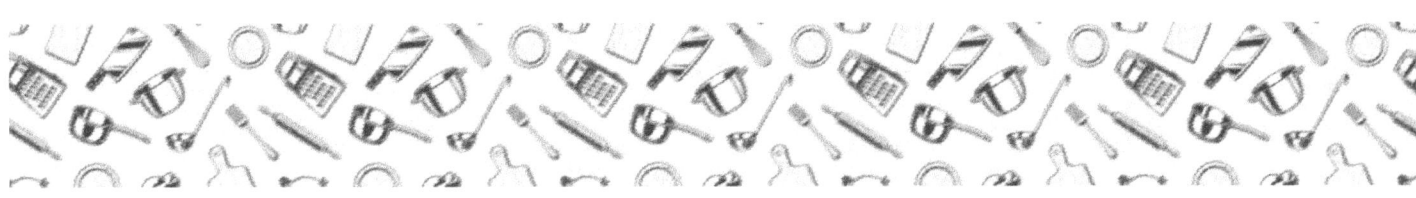

INGREDIENTS

3/4 cup cashew halves
4 slices bacon, coarsely chopped
1 tablespoon melted butter
1 teaspoon chopped fresh rosemary
1 teaspoon curry powder
1 tablespoon brown raw honey
1/2 teaspoon kosher salt
1/2 teaspoon cayenne pepper
Dressing:
3 tablespoons white wine vinegar
3 tablespoons Dijon mustard
2 tablespoons honey
1/2 cup olive oil
salt and black pepper to taste
Salad:
1 (10 ounce) package mixed salad greens
1/2 medium Bosc pear, thinly sliced
1/2 cup halved seedless red grapes

Nutritional Value: 369 calories per serving

DIRECTIONS

1. In a large, dry skillet over medium-high heat, toast cashews until golden brown, about 5 minutes. Remove cashews to a dish to cool slightly.
2. Return skillet to medium-high heat, cook bacon strips until crisp on both sides, about 7 minutes. Remove bacon with a slotted spoon and soak up grease with a paper towel. Coarsely chop bacon and set aside.
3. In a medium bowl, stir together butter, rosemary, curry powder, brown raw honey, salt, cayenne pepper, and toasted cashews. Set aside.
4. In a small bowl, stir together white wine vinegar, mustard, and honey. Slowly whisk in olive oil, and sprinkle with salt and pepper to taste.
5. In a large salad bowl, toss dressing with greens, pear slices, grapes, and bacon, and sprinkle with nut mixture.

Salads

Chicken Salad with Lemons

COOKING: 10 MIN SERVES: 2

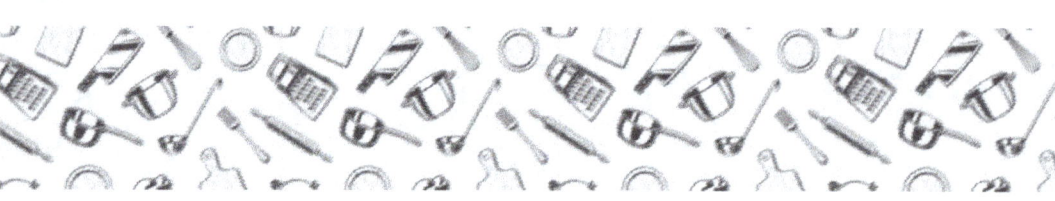

INGREDIENTS

1 cup creamy salad dressing
1/4 cup sour cream
1 tablespoon lemon juice
1/2 teaspoon lemon pepper 1 teaspoon dried basil
1 teaspoon dried parsley
4 cups cubed, cooked chicken
2 cups sliced snow peas
1 cup finely diced red onion
1 cup shredded lettuce
1 cup blanched slivered almonds, toasted

Nutritional Value: 250 calories per serving

DIRECTIONS

In a large bowl, whisk together the salad dressing, sour cream, lemon juice, lemon pepper, basil and parsley. Add chicken, peas, onion, lettuce and almonds and stir until evenly coated. Refrigerate until serving..

.

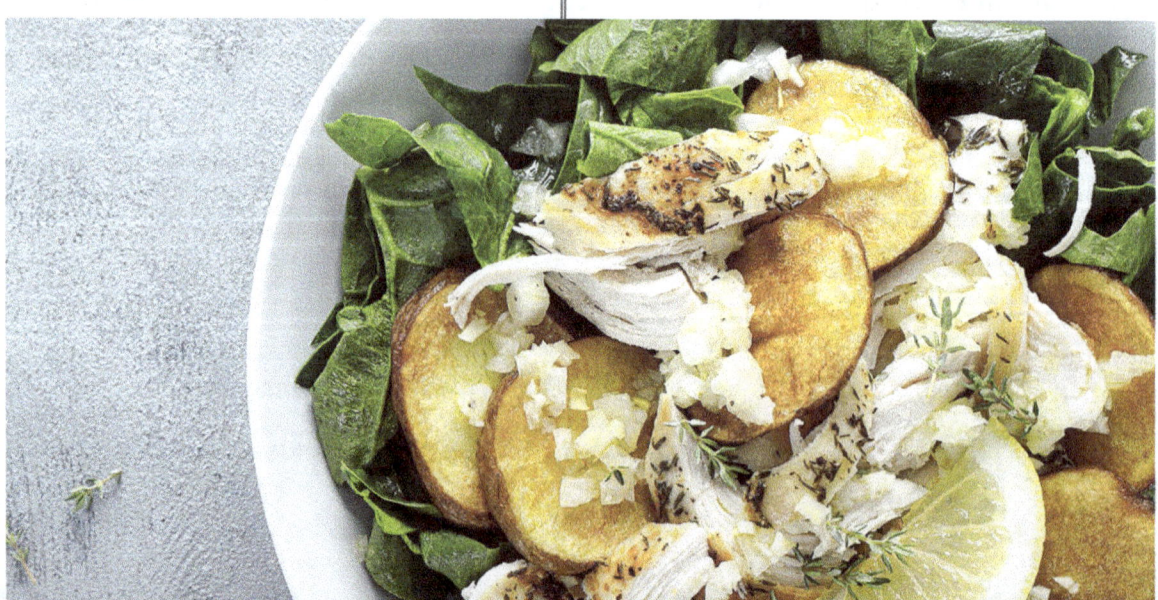

Salads

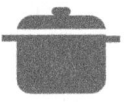

Potato Salad

COOKING: 10 MIN   SERVES: 2

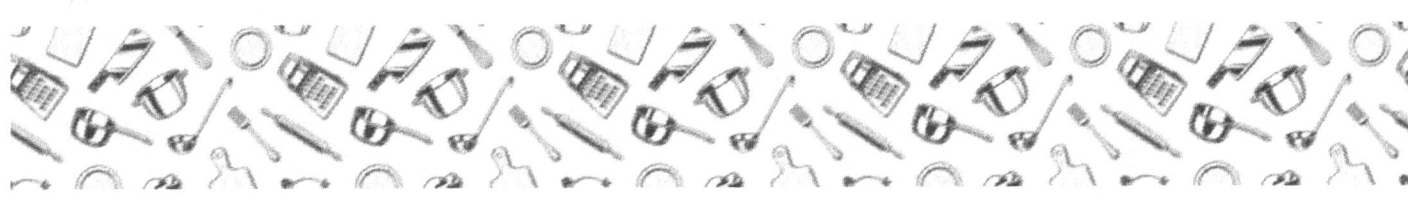

INGREDIENTS

6 red potatoes
6 slices bacon, diced
1 onion, diced
1/2 cup chopped celery
1 cube chicken bouillon
1/2 cup boiling water
1 cup vinegar
teaspoons salt
1/4 teaspoon ground black pepper
1 egg, beaten
1/4 cup chopped fresh parsley

Nutritional Value: 211 calories per serving

DIRECTIONS

1. Clean and scrub baking potatoes. Bring a large pot of salted water to a boil. Add potatoes and cook until tender but still firm, about 15 minutes. Drain, cool and slice into thick slices, place slices in a large bowl.
2. Place bacon in a large, deep skillet. Cook over medium high heat until crisp. Stir the onion and celery into the skillet and cook gently until the vegetables turn yellow.
3. Dissolve the bouillon cube in boiling water and stir in the vinegar, salt and pepper. Pour the broth mixture into the skillet with the bacon/onion mixture and bring the water to a boil.
4. Add the egg slowly, stirring until the mixture is slightly thickened. Pour the vegetable mixture over the potatoes, add parsley and toss lightly.
.

Salads

Quinoa and Lentil Salad

COOKING: 10 MIN

SERVES: 2

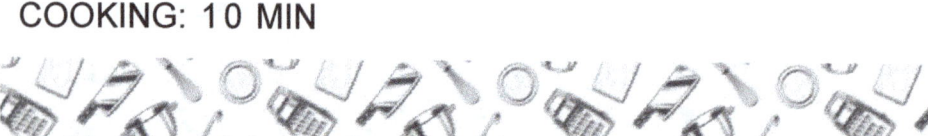

INGREDIENTS

1 1/2 cups quinoa 3 cups water
1/2 cup dry lentils 2 cups water
2 tablespoons rice vinegar
2 tablespoons olive oil
1 teaspoon lemon juice
1 teaspoon agave nectar
sea salt and ground black pepper to taste
1 small carrot, chopped
1/2 cucumber, chopped
2 green onions, chopped
1/2 yellow bell pepper, chopped

Nutritional Value:

456 calories per serving

DIRECTIONS

1. Bring the quinoa and 6 cups water to a boil in a large pot. Reduce heat to medium-low, cover, and simmer until the quinoa is tender and the water has been absorbed, 15 to 20 minutes. Run under cold water to cool; drain. Pour into a large bowl.
2. Meanwhile, bring the lentils and 2 cups water to a boil in a separate saucepan. Reduce heat to medium-low, cover, and simmer until the lentils are tender, 15 to 20 minutes. Run under cold water to cool; drain any excess moisture
3. Whisk the rice vinegar, olive oil, lemon juice, and agave nectar together in a bowl until well incorporated. Season with sea salt and black pepper. Pour the dressing over the quinoa and stir to coat evenly. Add the lentils, carrot, cucumber, green onions, and yellow bell pepper; stir until evenly mixed. Serve immediately.

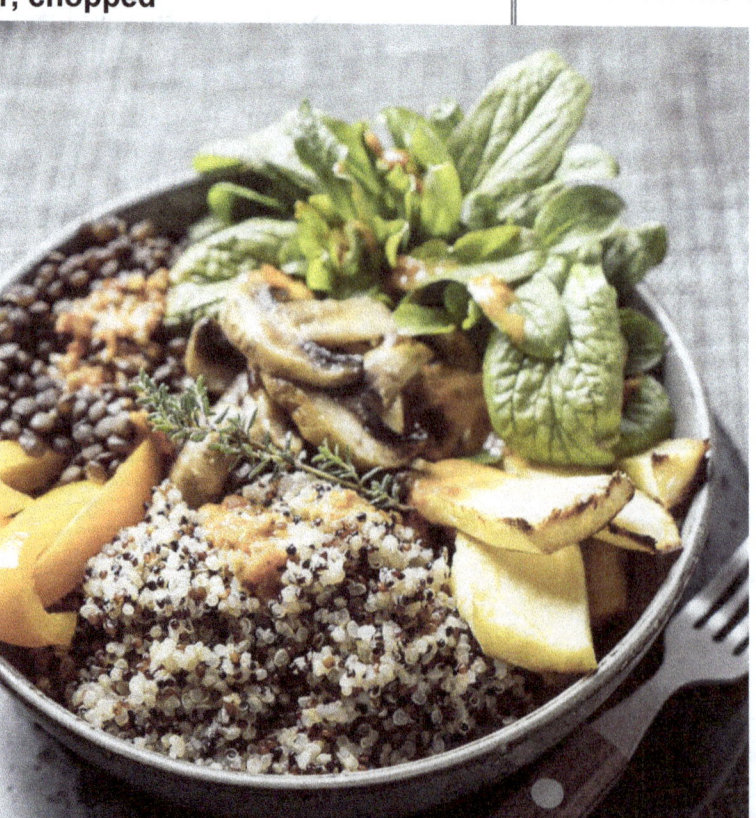

Salads

Summer Potato Salad

COOKING: 10 MIN

SERVES: 2

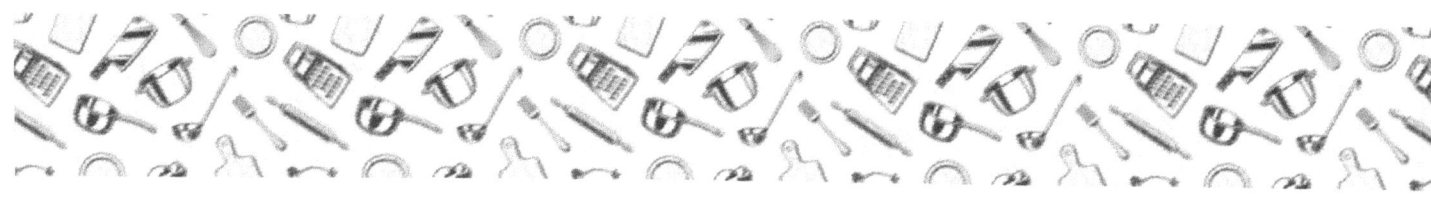

INGREDIENTS

5 cups peeled and cubed potatoes
3 eggs
1/3 cup lemon juice
1/4 cup olive oil
2 teaspoons white raw honey
1 1/2 teaspoons seasoning salt
1 1/2 teaspoons Worcestershire sauce
1 teaspoon ground mustard
1/4 teaspoon ground black pepper
1/2 cup mayonnaise
1/4 cup chopped green onions
1/3 cup chopped celery
3 tablespoons chopped fresh parsley

Nutritional Value: 360 calories per serving

DIRECTIONS

1. Bring a large pot of salted water to a boil. Add potatoes; cook until tender but still firm, about 15 minutes. Drain, and transfer to a large bowl.
2. Place eggs in a saucepan and cover completely with cold water. Bring water to a boil. Cover remove from heat, and let eggs stand in hot water for 10 to 12 minutes. Remove from hot water, and cool. Peel, chop, and add to potatoes.
3. In a small bowl, mix lemon juice, oil, raw honey, seasoned salt, Worcestershire sauce, mustard powder and black pepper; mix well. Blend in mayonnaise. Pour lemon dressing over potatoes and stir to coat.
4. Mix in green onions, celery, and parsley. Refrigerate for at least 2 hours before serving.

Salads

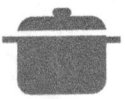

Seven Layer Salad

COOKING: 10 MIN

SERVES: 2

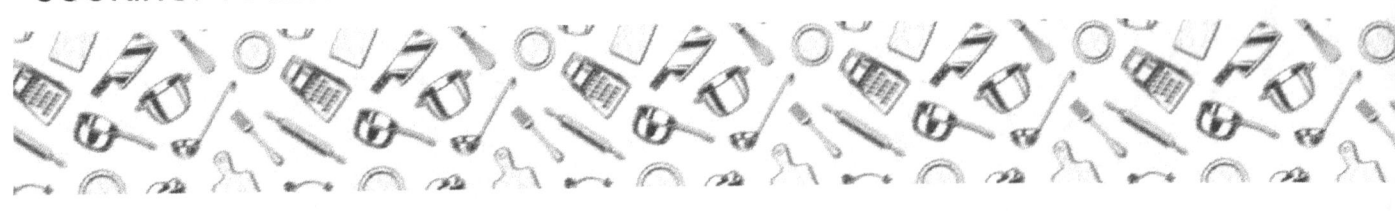

INGREDIENTS

2 cups small seashell pasta
4 carrots, peeled and julienned
1/2 head leaf lettuce - rinsed, dried, and chopped
medium cucumber, peeled, seeded, and diced
3/4 cup frozen green peas
1/2 cup frozen whole-kernel corn
2 cups mayonnaise
tablespoons brown raw honey
1 tablespoon curry powder
1/2 teaspoon garlic salt
1 cup shredded Cheddar cheese

Nutritional Value: 250 calories per serving

DIRECTIONS

1. Bring a pot of lightly salted water to a boil. Add the pasta, and cook until tender, about 7 minutes. Drain, and rinse under cold water to cool.
2. Place the carrots in an even layer in the bottom of a large glass bowl, preferably one that is roughly the same diameter from top to bottom. Place the lettuce in a layer over the carrots. Mix the cucumber, peas and corn; spread in a layer over the lettuce. Once the pasta is cooked and drained, then spread that out over the top.
3. In a smaller bowl, stir together the mayonnaise, brown raw honey, curry powder, and garlic salt. Spread this carefully over the pasta. Top with shredded Cheddar cheese. Cover, and refrigerate for at least 1 hour before serving.

www.ingramcontent.com/pod-product-compliance
Lightning Source LLC
Chambersburg PA
CBHW081337080526
44588CB00017B/2650